DASH DIET FOR BEGINNERS

The Complete Guide to Help Prevent or Improve High Blood Pressure and Preserve Your Heart Health. Easy Delicious Nutrition Budget-Friendly Recipes. 30-day Meal Plan

Emma Willson

Copyright © 2023 by Emma Willson

Disclaimer:

The information provided in this cookbook is for general informational purposes only and does not constitute professional medical advice. The DASH Diet cookbook is not intended to diagnose, treat, cure, or prevent any medical condition. Always seek the advice of your physician or other qualified health provider with any questions you may have regarding a medical condition.

The recipes and dietary suggestions presented in this cookbook are based on general principles of healthy eating and the DASH Diet guidelines. However, individual nutritional needs may vary, and it is essential to consult with a healthcare professional or a registered dietitian before making significant changes to your diet, especially if you have any pre-existing health conditions.

The authors and publishers of this cookbook are not responsible for any adverse effects or consequences resulting from using the information contained herein. Readers are encouraged to use their judgment and seek professional advice as needed.

While every effort has been made to ensure the accuracy and completeness of the information provided, the authors and publishers cannot be held responsible for any errors or omissions. Product availability and nutritional information may also change over time, and the reader must verify this information independently.

By using this cookbook, you acknowledge and agree to the terms of this disclaimer.

Table of contents

INTRODUCTION

Welcome to the "Dash Diet Cookbook" – your guide to the world of delicious and healthy dishes crafted by the principles of the DASH diet. This book invites you on a culinary journey focusing on your health and well-being.

DASH (Dietary Approaches to Stop Hypertension) is not just a diet; it's a lifestyle promoting lowering blood pressure and improving cardiovascular health. In this book, we offer recipes that align with the principles of the DASH diet and culinary ideas that will make your meals diverse, flavorful, and nutritious.

Why the DASH Diet?

The DASH diet balances satisfying your taste buds and supporting your health. It emphasizes consuming nutrient-rich foods such as fruits, vegetables, low-fat dairy products, nuts, and whole grains while limiting salt intake. Our book aims to make the DASH diet tasty and accessible, even if you're not an experienced chef.

What Will You Find in the "Dash Diet Cookbook"?

Within the pages of this book, you'll discover over 100 innovative and delightful recipes specifically designed to satisfy your palate and add variety to your table. From hearty breakfasts to delectable desserts, each recipe in our book adheres to the principles of the DASH diet, ensuring balance and healthfulness.

Embark on the Journey to Better Health!

Join us on this tasty and beneficial journey. Together, let's explore the world of health and inspiration in cooking, where each meal becomes an opportunity to care for your body. The "Dash Diet Cookbook" is your reliable companion on the path to a healthy lifestyle and superb taste!

Chapter 1. UNDERSTANDING THE DASH DIET

The DASH Diet, an acronym for Dietary Approaches to Stop Hypertension, is rooted in research funded by the US National Institute of Health (NIH). This research aimed to uncover the impact of diet on blood pressure. The DASH program was subsequently designed to provide a flavorful and balanced alternative for individuals with high blood pressure. It offers more than just a dietary approach—it's a pathway to better health.

The primary goal of the DASH diet is to lower high blood pressure, as its name suggests. According to the NIH, it goes beyond merely managing blood pressure; it promotes healthy eating habits, steering individuals away from processed and junk foods. The focus is on reducing salt intake while increasing the consumption of essential nutrients like calcium, magnesium, and potassium.

Beyond its impact on blood pressure, the DASH diet has proven effective in reducing the risk of various health issues, including cardiovascular disease, certain cancers, stroke, diabetes, heart disease, kidney disease, and heart failure. Recognized for its simplicity and sustainability, the DASH diet has consistently earned accolades. It has been named the best diet for overall health and the top diabetes diet by the US News & World Report for consecutive years.

While weight loss wasn't the primary aim of the DASH diet, its emphasis on mindful calorie consumption and healthy foods naturally leads to shedding pounds. This unintended yet beneficial outcome is particularly advantageous for overweight individuals dealing with hypertension. With the DASH diet, achieving a weight loss of 2 kilograms per week becomes feasible and relatively effortless, offering an additional incentive for those looking to manage their blood pressure effectively.

Phases of the DASH Diet

The DASH Diet unfolds in two distinct phases, each tailored to promote optimal health and well-being.

1. Salt Reduction Phases:

   - The initial research-backed DASH diet recommendations involve a two-phase approach to salt reduction.

   - In Phase 1, salt intake is capped at 2300mg daily, equivalent to a teaspoon.

   - Phase 2 further restricts salt to 1500mg daily, eliminating table salt entirely, even when dining out or consuming packaged foods.

   - Recognizing that salt and sodium are often used interchangeably, it's crucial to note that salt is a primary source of dietary sodium.

2. Weight Management Phases:

- Phase 1 of the DASH Diet initiates a two-week low-carb phase, excluding fruits and whole grains. This phase aims to enhance natural calorie-burning mechanisms and reset metabolism, leading to rapid and visible weight loss.

- The focus is on developing sustainable eating habits for life, controlling blood sugar levels, and reducing hunger. During Phase 1, individuals abstain from fruits, whole grains, and alcohol while incorporating low-fat dairy and lean protein sources such as fish, nuts, and lean meats.

- Emphasizing non-starchy vegetable proteins and eliminating grains and sugar, Phase 1 helps regulate insulin levels, making individuals crave lighter, healthier meals.

- Nutrient-rich options like leafy greens and cruciferous vegetables such as broccoli, cabbage, and cauliflower; cucumbers, peppers, tomatoes, squash, seeds, nuts, and fatty seafood become integral to this phase.

- Phase 2 extends the benefits of Phase 1, emphasizing heart-healthy choices by excluding starchy vegetables. The green light is given to fish, lean meats, fruits, and vegetables, resulting in weight loss and reduced blood cholesterol.

With its dual focus on salt reduction and weight management, the DASH Diet offers a structured and practical approach to achieving both heart health and overall well-being.

Starting with The DASH Diet

Embarking on the DASH Diet doesn't require drastic changes overnight. Instead, ease into it by making minor adjustments that align with your preferences. Consider the following approach:

- Incorporate one serving of vegetables or fruits into each meal.

- Experiment with 2 or more meatless meals weekly.

- Opt for spices and herbs over salt for added flavor.

- Swap chips for a healthier alternative like almonds or nuts.

- Substitute white flour with whole-wheat flour when possible.

- Take a 15-minute stroll after lunch or dinner, or both.

Benefits of the DASH Diet

While we've explored the DASH diet and its noteworthy advantages for daily living, let's delve deeper into its specific benefits.

1. High Blood Pressure Prevention and Treatment

The DASH diet offers a healthy alternative for many in the U.S. relying on blood pressure medication. Lowering blood pressure reduces the risk of heart disease, strokes, kidney disease, and heart attacks. The National Institutes of Health (NIH) notes that adhering to the DASH diet for ten years could potentially prevent around 400,000 cardiovascular disease-related deaths, significantly improving overall population health.

2. Treatment and Prevention of Metabolic Syndrome

The DASH diet positively influences blood pressure, blood sugar, triglycerides, bad cholesterol, and insulin resistance. For individuals dealing with metabolic syndrome, obesity, or type 2 diabetes, this dietary approach proves beneficial. Changes in blood pressure and systolic pressure can be observed within weeks. Additionally, the DASH diet has demonstrated a capacity to lower the risk of colorectal cancer, offering a potentially life-saving remedy for common health issues.

3. Getting in Shape

While the primary focus of the DASH diet isn't necessarily weight loss, it can be a positive side effect. The diet naturally avoids weight gain triggers, such as sweets and red meat. Adjustments like reducing poultry and fish while increasing vegetable intake can contribute to healthy weight loss. Moreover, breaking away from the conventional three-meals-a-day rule allows your metabolism to work more efficiently, aiding in weight loss.

4. Immune System Strengthening

Rich in antioxidants, the DASH diet includes foods that assist your body in producing antioxidants to protect cells from free radicals. Strengthening the immune system helps guard against severe diseases like cancer and heart disease. This becomes especially crucial during flu season.

Chapter 1. BREAKFAST

Quinoa and Vegetable Power Bowl

Ingredients:
- 1 cup quinoa (200g)

- 2 cups mixed vegetables (broccoli, bell peppers, carrots) (300g)

- 1 tablespoon olive oil (15ml)

- 1 teaspoon lemon juice (5ml)

- Salt and pepper to taste

Instructions:
1. Cook quinoa according to package instructions.

2. In a pan, sauté mixed vegetables in olive oil until tender.

3. Mix cooked quinoa and sautéed vegetables.

4. Drizzle with lemon juice and season with salt and pepper.

5. Serve warm.

Nutrition:
Calories: 350 | Protein: 12g | Carbs: 55g | Fat: 10g | Fiber: 8g

Prep time: 10 minutes | Cook time: 20 minutes | Servings: 2

Berry and Greek Yogurt Parfait

Ingredients:
- 1 cup Greek yogurt (240g)

- 1/2 cup mixed berries (blueberries, strawberries) (75g)

- 2 tablespoons granola (30g)

- 1 tablespoon honey (15ml)

Instructions:
1. Layer Greek yogurt, mixed berries, and granola in a glass.

2. Drizzle honey on top.

3. Repeat layers.

4. Top with a few berries.

5. Enjoy!

Nutrition:
Calories: 280 | Protein: 15g | Carbs: 45g | Fat: 5g | Fiber: 6g

Prep time: 5 minutes | Cook time: 0 minutes | Servings: 1

Spinach and Feta Egg Muffins

Ingredients:
- 6 eggs

- 1 cup fresh spinach, chopped (30g)

- 1/2 cup feta cheese, crumbled (75g)

- Salt and pepper to taste

Instructions:
1. Preheat oven to 350°F (180°C).

2. In a bowl, whisk eggs.

3. Add chopped spinach, feta, salt, and pepper.

4. Pour mixture into a greased muffin tin.

5. Bake for 15-20 minutes or until eggs are set.

6. Serve warm.

Nutrition:
Calories: 220 | Protein: 18g | Carbs: 2g | Fat: 15g | Fiber: 1g

Prep time: 10 minutes | Cook time: 15-20 minutes | Servings: 3

Avocado Toast Extravaganza

Ingredients:
- 2 slices whole-grain bread

- 1 ripe avocado

- 1 tablespoon olive oil (15ml)

- Salt and pepper to taste

- Red pepper flakes (optional)

Instructions:
1. Toast the whole-grain bread slices.

2. Mash the ripe avocado and spread it evenly on the toast.

3. Drizzle with olive oil and season with salt and pepper.

4. Sprinkle red pepper flakes if desired.

5. Serve immediately.

Nutrition:
Calories: 280 | Protein: 6g | Carbs: 25g | Fat: 18g | Fiber: 10g

Prep time: 5 minutes | Cook time: 5 minutes | Servings: 1

Zesty Tomato and Basil Frittata

Ingredients:
- 4 eggs

- 1 cup cherry tomatoes, halved (150g)

- 1/4 cup fresh basil, chopped (10g)

- 1/2 cup feta cheese, crumbled (75g)

- Salt and pepper to taste

Instructions:
1. Preheat oven to 350°F (180°C).

2. In a bowl, whisk eggs.

3. Add halved cherry tomatoes, chopped basil, crumbled feta, salt, and pepper.

4. Pour the mixture into a greased baking dish.

5. Bake for 20-25 minutes or until the frittata is set.

6. Slice and serve.

Nutrition:
Calories: 320 | Protein: 18g | Carbs: 8g | Fat: 24g | Fiber: 2g

Prep time: 10 minutes | Cook time: 20-25 minutes | Servings: 2

Cinnamon Apple Oatmeal Elegance

Ingredients:
- 1 cup rolled oats (100g)

- 1 cup almond milk (240ml)

- 1 apple, diced

- 1 teaspoon cinnamon

- 1 tablespoon maple syrup (15ml)

- Chopped nuts for garnish (optional)

Instructions:
1. In a saucepan, combine rolled oats and almond milk. Cook over medium heat.

2. Add diced apple, cinnamon, and maple syrup. Stir well.

3. Cook until oats are tender and the mixture thickens.

4. Garnish with chopped nuts if desired.

5. Serve warm.

Nutrition:
Calories: 320 | Protein: 8g | Carbs: 60g | Fat: 6g | Fiber: 10g

Prep time: 5 minutes | Cook time: 10 minutes | Servings: 1

Smoked Salmon and Cream Cheese Bagel

Ingredients:
- 1 whole-grain bagel

- 2 ounces smoked salmon (60g)

- 2 tablespoons cream cheese (30g)

- Sliced cucumber and red onion for topping

Instructions:
1. Toast the whole-grain bagel to your liking.

2. Spread cream cheese on each bagel half.

3. Layer smoked salmon on top of the cream cheese.

4. Add sliced cucumber and red onion for extra flavor.

5. Assemble the bagel and enjoy.

Nutrition:
Calories: 350 | Protein: 20g | Carbs: 45g | Fat: 12g | Fiber: 5g

Prep time: 5 minutes | Cook time: 5 minutes | Servings: 1

Sweet Potato Hash Sunrise

Ingredients:
- 1 sweet potato, peeled and diced

- 1/2 onion, diced

- 1 bell pepper, diced

- 2 tablespoons olive oil (30ml)

- 1 teaspoon paprika

- Salt and pepper to taste

- Poached eggs for topping

Instructions:
1. In a skillet, heat olive oil over medium heat.

2. Add diced sweet potato, onion, and bell pepper.

3. Sprinkle with paprika, salt, and pepper.

4. Cook until the sweet potato is tender and the vegetables are golden.

5. Top with poached eggs.

6. Serve warm.

Nutrition:
Calories: 320 | Protein: 12g | Carbs: 40g | Fat: 15g | Fiber: 7g

Prep time: 10 minutes | Cook time: 15 minutes | Servings: 2

Tropical Fruit Smoothie Bowl

Ingredients:
- 1 cup frozen mixed tropical fruits (pineapple, mango, banana) (150g)

- 1/2 cup Greek yogurt (120g)

- 1/4 cup granola (30g)

- Coconut flakes and chia seeds for topping

Instructions:
1. Blend frozen fruits and Greek yogurt until smooth.

2. Pour into a bowl.

3. Top with granola, coconut flakes, and chia seeds.

4. Enjoy with a spoon.

Nutrition:
Calories: 280 | Protein: 10g | Carbs: 45g | Fat: 7g | Fiber: 6g

Prep time: 5 minutes | Cook time: 0 minutes | Servings: 1

Whole Wheat Pancake Perfection

Ingredients:
- 1 cup whole wheat flour (120g)

- 1 tablespoon baking powder (15g)

- 1 tablespoon honey (15ml)

- 1 cup almond milk (240ml)

- 1 egg

- Fresh berries for topping

Instructions:
1. Whisk together whole wheat flour, baking powder, honey, almond milk, and egg in a bowl.

2. Heat a griddle or non-stick pan over medium heat.

3. Pour batter onto the griddle to form pancakes.

4. Cook until bubbles form on the surface, then flip and cook the other side.

5. Serve topped with fresh berries.

Nutrition:
Calories: 280 | Protein: 9g | Carbs: 45g | Fat: 7g | Fiber: 6g

Prep time: 10 minutes | Cook time: 10 minutes | Servings: 2

Mediterranean Veggie Scramble

Ingredients:
- 4 eggs

- 1/2 cup cherry tomatoes, halved (75g)

- 1/4 cup black olives, sliced (30g)

- 1/4 cup feta cheese, crumbled (30g)

- Fresh oregano for garnish

Instructions:
1. In a bowl, whisk eggs.

2. Heat a skillet over medium heat.

3. Add cherry tomatoes, black olives, and crumbled feta to the skillet.

4. Pour whisked eggs over the vegetables and scramble.

5. Cook until eggs are set.

6. Garnish with fresh oregano.

7. Serve hot.

Nutrition:
Calories: 320 | Protein: 18g | Carbs: 6g | Fat: 24g | Fiber: 2g

Prep time: 10 minutes | Cook time: 10 minutes | Servings: 2

Blueberry Almond Breakfast Quinoa

Ingredients:
- 1 cup cooked quinoa (200g)

- 1/2 cup almond milk (120ml)

- 1/2 cup fresh blueberries (75g)

- 1 tablespoon almond butter (15g)

- 1 teaspoon maple syrup (5ml)

Instructions:

1. In a bowl, mix cooked quinoa and almond milk.

2. Gently fold in fresh blueberries.

3. Drizzle with almond butter and maple syrup.

4. Stir well and serve.

Nutrition:

Calories: 320 | Protein: 10g | Carbs: 50g | Fat: 10g | Fiber: 8g

Prep time: 5 minutes | Cook time: 5 minutes | Servings: 1

Green Goddess Breakfast Wrap

Ingredients:

- 1 whole-grain wrap

- 2 eggs, scrambled

- Handful of baby spinach

- 1/4 avocado, sliced

- Salsa for topping

Instructions:

1. Cook scrambled eggs in a pan.

2. Lay out the whole-grain wrap.

3. Place scrambled eggs, baby spinach, and sliced avocado on the wrap.

4. Top with salsa.

5. Fold the wrap and serve.

Nutrition:

Calories: 340 | Protein: 15g | Carbs: 25g | Fat: 20g | Fiber: 8g

Prep time: 10 minutes | Cook time: 5 minutes | Servings: 1

Almond Butter Banana Toast

Ingredients:

- 2 slices whole-grain bread

- 2 tablespoons almond butter (30g)

- 1 banana, sliced

- Drizzle of honey (optional)

Instructions:
1. Toast the whole-grain bread slices.

2. Spread almond butter on each slice.

3. Arrange banana slices on top.

4. Drizzle with honey if desired.

5. Enjoy!

Nutrition:
Calories: 300 | Protein: 8g | Carbs: 45g | Fat: 12g | Fiber: 8g

Prep time: 5 minutes | Cook time: 5 minutes | Servings: 1

Protein-Packed Cottage Cheese Parfait

Ingredients:
- 1 cup low-fat cottage cheese (240g)

- 1/2 cup mixed berries (blueberries, raspberries) (75g)

- 2 tablespoons granola (30g)

- 1 tablespoon honey (15ml)

Instructions:
1. Layer low-fat cottage cheese, mixed berries, and granola in a glass.

2. Drizzle honey on top.

3. Repeat layers.

4. Enjoy with a spoon.

Nutrition:
Calories: 280 | Protein: 20g | Carbs: 30g | Fat: 8g | Fiber: 5g

Prep time: 5 minutes | Cook time: 0 minutes | Servings: 1

Mushroom and Spinach Breakfast Burrito

Ingredients:
- 2 whole eggs, scrambled

- 1/2 cup mushrooms, sliced (75g)

- 1 cup fresh spinach leaves (30g)

- 1 whole-grain tortilla

- Salsa for topping

Instructions:
1. In a pan, cook scrambled eggs until fluffy.

2. Add sliced mushrooms and fresh spinach to the pan.

3. Cook until the vegetables are tender.

4. Warm the whole-grain tortilla.

5. Fill the tortilla with the egg and vegetable mixture.

6. Top with salsa.

7. Roll into a burrito and serve.

Nutrition:
Calories: 320 | Protein: 18g | Carbs: 30g | Fat: 15g | Fiber: 7g

Prep time: 10 minutes | Cook time: 10 minutes | Servings: 1

Cranberry Walnut Overnight Oats

Ingredients:
- 1/2 cup rolled oats (50g)

- 1/2 cup almond milk (120ml)

- 2 tablespoons dried cranberries (30g)

- 1 tablespoon chopped walnuts (15g)

- 1 teaspoon honey (5ml)

Instructions:
1. In a jar, combine rolled oats and almond milk.

2. Add dried cranberries and chopped walnuts.

3. Drizzle with honey.

4. Stir well, cover, and refrigerate overnight.

5. Enjoy chilled.

Nutrition:
Calories: 290 | Protein: 7g | Carbs: 40g | Fat: 12g | Fiber: 6g

Prep time: 5 minutes | Cook time: 0 minutes | Servings: 1

Tomato Basil Breakfast Sandwich

Ingredients:
- 1 whole-grain English muffin

- 1 large egg, fried

- 1 slice tomato

- Fresh basil leaves

- Salt and pepper to taste

Instructions:
1. Toast the whole-grain English muffin.

2. Fry the egg to your liking.

3. Assemble the sandwich with the egg, tomato slice, and fresh basil.

4. Season with salt and pepper.

5. Serve immediately.

Nutrition:
Calories: 250 | Protein: 14g | Carbs: 30g | Fat: 10g | Fiber: 5g

Prep time: 5 minutes | Cook time: 5 minutes | Servings: 1

Greek Yogurt and Berry Pancake Stack

Ingredients:
- 2 whole-grain pancakes

- 1/2 cup Greek yogurt (120g)

- Mixed berries (blueberries, strawberries) for topping (75g)

- 1 tablespoon honey (15ml)

Instructions:
1. Stack the whole-grain pancakes on a plate.

2. Spread Greek yogurt over each pancake.

3. Top with mixed berries.

4. Drizzle honey over the stack.

5. Enjoy this delightful pancake treat!

Nutrition:
Calories: 280 | Protein: 10g | Carbs: 50g | Fat: 5g | Fiber: 6g

Prep time: 10 minutes | Cook time: 10 minutes | Servings: 1

Southwest Quinoa Breakfast Skillet

Ingredients:
- 1 cup cooked quinoa (200g)

- 1/2 cup black beans, drained and rinsed (75g)

- 1/4 cup corn kernels (30g)

- 1/4 cup diced bell peppers (30g)

- 1/4 cup salsa

- 1/2 avocado, sliced

Instructions:
1. Combine cooked quinoa, black beans, corn, and diced bell peppers in a skillet.

2. Stir in salsa and cook until heated through.

3. Top with sliced avocado.

4. Serve warm.

Nutrition:
Calories: 350 | Protein: 12g | Carbs: 50g | Fat: 12g | Fiber: 10g

Prep time: 10 minutes | Cook time: 10 minutes | Servings: 2

Pear and Walnut Breakfast Salad

Ingredients:
- 1 pear, thinly sliced

- 1/4 cup walnuts, chopped (30g)

- 1 cup mixed salad greens (spinach, arugula)

- 1 tablespoon balsamic vinaigrette dressing (15ml)

Instructions:
1. In a bowl, toss together sliced pear, chopped walnuts, and mixed salad greens.

2. Drizzle with balsamic vinaigrette dressing.

3. Gently toss until well combined.

4. Serve this refreshing breakfast salad.

Nutrition:
Calories: 260 | Protein: 5g | Carbs: 30g | Fat: 15g | Fiber: 6g

Prep time: 10 minutes | Cook time: 0 minutes | Servings: 1

Chickpea and Spinach Breakfast Hash

Ingredients:
- 1 can (15 oz) chickpeas, drained and rinsed

- 2 cups fresh spinach leaves (60g)

- 1/2 red onion, diced

- 1 bell pepper, diced

- 2 tablespoons olive oil (30ml)

- 1 teaspoon smoked paprika

- Salt and pepper to taste

Instructions:
1. In a skillet, heat olive oil over medium heat.

2. Add diced red onion and bell pepper. Sauté until softened.

3. Stir in chickpeas and smoked paprika.

4. Add fresh spinach and cook until wilted.

5. Season with salt and pepper.

6. Serve warm.

Nutrition:
Calories: 320 | Protein: 12g | Carbs: 40g | Fat: 15g | Fiber: 10g

Prep time: 10 minutes | Cook time: 15 minutes | Servings: 2

Orange and Pistachio Chia Pudding

Ingredients:
- 1/4 cup chia seeds (40g)

- 1 cup almond milk (240ml)

- Zest and juice of 1 orange

- 1 tablespoon chopped pistachios (15g)

- 1 teaspoon honey (5ml)

Instructions:
1. In a bowl, mix chia seeds and almond milk.

2. Add orange zest and juice, chopped pistachios, and honey.

3. Stir well, cover, and refrigerate for at least 2 hours or overnight.

4. Before serving, stir the pudding and top with additional pistachios.

5. Enjoy!

Nutrition:
Calories: 280 | Protein: 8g | Carbs: 30g | Fat: 15g | Fiber: 12g

Prep time: 5 minutes | Cook time: 2 hours (chilling) | Servings: 1

Turkey Sausage and Veggie Egg Cups

Ingredients:
- 4 eggs

- 1/2 cup turkey sausage, cooked and crumbled (75g)

- 1/2 cup mixed vegetables (bell peppers, spinach) (75g)

- Salt and pepper to taste

Instructions:
1. Preheat oven to 350°F (180°C).

2. In a bowl, whisk eggs.

3. Stir in cooked turkey sausage and mixed vegetables.

4. Pour the mixture into greased muffin tin cups.

5. Bake for 15-20 minutes or until eggs are set.

6. Serve warm.

Nutrition:
Calories: 280 | Protein: 18g | Carbs: 6g | Fat: 20g | Fiber: 2g

Prep time: 10 minutes | Cook time: 15-20 minutes | Servings: 2

Banana Nut Overnight Oats

Ingredients:
- 1/2 cup rolled oats (50g)

- 1/2 cup almond milk (120ml)

- 1 ripe banana, mashed

- 1 tablespoon chopped nuts (walnuts, almonds) (15g)

- 1 teaspoon honey (5ml)

Instructions:
1. In a jar, combine rolled oats and almond milk.

2. Add mashed ripe banana and chopped nuts.

3. Drizzle with honey.

4. Stir well, cover, and refrigerate overnight.

5. Enjoy this delicious and nutritious breakfast!

Nutrition:
Calories: 280 | Protein: 8g | Carbs: 45g | Fat: 8g | Fiber: 7g

Prep time: 5 minutes | Cook time: 0 minutes (overnight) | Servings: 1

Pesto and Tomato Breakfast Wrap

Ingredients:
- 1 whole-grain wrap

- 2 eggs, scrambled

- 1 tablespoon pesto sauce (15g)

- Cherry tomatoes, halved

- Salt and pepper to taste

Instructions:
1. Cook scrambled eggs in a pan.

2. Lay out the whole-grain wrap.

3. Spread pesto sauce on the wrap.

4. Add scrambled eggs and halved cherry tomatoes.

5. Season with salt and pepper.

6. Roll into a wrap and serve.

Nutrition:
Calories: 320 | Protein: 18g | Carbs: 25g | Fat: 18g | Fiber: 5g

Prep time: 10 minutes | Cook time: 5 minutes | Servings: 1

Cacao and Almond Butter Smoothie

Ingredients:
- 1 cup almond milk (240ml)

- 1 banana

- 1 tablespoon almond butter (15g)

- 1 tablespoon cacao powder (15g)

- Ice cubes (optional)

Instructions:
1. Combine almond milk, banana, almond butter, and cacao powder in a blender.

2. Blend until smooth.

3. Add ice cubes if desired and blend again.

4. Pour into a glass and enjoy this chocolatey smoothie!

Nutrition:
Calories: 300 | Protein: 7g | Carbs: 40g | Fat: 15g | Fiber: 8g

Prep time: 5 minutes | Cook time: 0 minutes | Servings: 1

Veggie-Packed Breakfast Burrito Bowl

Ingredients:
- 1/2 cup cooked quinoa (100g)

- 1/2 cup black beans, drained and rinsed (75g)

- 1/2 cup sautéed bell peppers and onions (75g)

- 1/4 cup salsa

- 1/4 avocado, sliced

- Fresh cilantro for garnish

Instructions:
1. In a bowl, layer cooked quinoa, black beans, sautéed bell peppers and onions.

2. Top with salsa and sliced avocado.

3. Garnish with fresh cilantro.

4. Mix before eating to combine all the flavors.

5. Enjoy this hearty and nutritious breakfast bowl!

Nutrition:
Calories: 330 | Protein: 12g | Carbs: 50g | Fat: 10g | Fiber: 12g

Prep time: 15 minutes | Cook time: 10 minutes | Servings: 1

Coconut Chia Seed Pudding Parfait

Ingredients:
- 2 tablespoons chia seeds (30g)

- 1/2 cup coconut milk (120ml)

- 1/4 cup granola (30g)

- 1/4 cup mixed berries (blueberries, raspberries) (40g)

- 1 tablespoon shredded coconut

Instructions:
1. In a jar, mix chia seeds and coconut milk.

2. Refrigerate for at least 2 hours or overnight.

3. Layer chia pudding, granola, and mixed berries in a glass.

4. Repeat layers and top with shredded coconut.

5. Dive into this delightful coconut chia seed parfait!

Nutrition:
Calories: 300 | Protein: 6g | Carbs: 40g | Fat: 15g | Fiber: 10g

Prep time: 5 minutes | Cook time: 2 hours (chilling) | Servings: 1

Apple Cinnamon Walnut Breakfast Bowl

Ingredients:
- 1 cup cooked steel-cut oats (200g)

- 1 apple, diced

- 1 tablespoon chopped walnuts (15g)

- 1 teaspoon cinnamon

- 1 teaspoon maple syrup (5ml)

Instructions:
1. Combine cooked steel-cut oats, diced apples, chopped walnuts, cinnamon, and maple syrup in a bowl.

2. Stir well.

3. Heat in the microwave if desired.

4. Savor the warmth of this apple cinnamon walnut breakfast bowl!

Nutrition:
Calories: 320 | Protein: 8g | Carbs: 50g | Fat: 10g | Fiber: 8g

Prep time: 10 minutes | Cook time: 5 minutes | Servings: 1

Grilled Chicken and Quinoa Salad

Ingredients:
- 2 boneless, skinless chicken breasts (about 225g each)

- 1 cup quinoa (200g)

- 2 cups cherry tomatoes, halved (400g)

- 1 cucumber, diced (about 150g)

- 1/4 cup red onion, finely chopped (25g)

- 1/4 cup feta cheese, crumbled (25g)

- 2 tablespoons olive oil (30ml)

- 1 tablespoon balsamic vinegar (15ml)

- Salt and black pepper to taste

Instructions:
1. Season chicken breasts with salt and black pepper.

2. Grill chicken until fully cooked, about 6-8 minutes per side. Allow it to rest before slicing.

3. Cook quinoa according to package instructions.

4. Combine quinoa, cherry tomatoes, cucumber, red onion, and feta cheese in a large bowl.

5. Whisk together olive oil and balsamic vinegar for the dressing.

6. Add sliced grilled chicken to the salad, drizzle with dressing, and toss gently.

7. Serve immediately.

Nutrition:
Calories - 480 | Protein - 35g | Carbs - 40g | Fat - 20g | Fiber - 6g

Prep time: 15 minutes | Cook time: 20 minutes | Servings: 2

Spinach and Feta Turkey Burger

Ingredients

- 1 pound ground turkey (450g)

- 1 cup fresh spinach, chopped (100g)

- 1/2 cup crumbled feta cheese (75g)

- 1/4 cup red onion, finely chopped (25g)

- 2 cloves garlic, minced

- 1 teaspoon dried oregano

- Salt and black pepper to taste

- Whole wheat burger buns

- Toppings: Lettuce, tomato slices, and tzatziki sauce

Instructions:

1. Preheat the grill or grill pan over medium-high heat.

2. Combine ground turkey, chopped spinach, crumbled feta cheese, red onion, minced garlic, dried oregano, salt, and black pepper in a large bowl.

3. Divide the mixture into equal portions and shape into burger patties.

4. Grill the turkey burgers for 5-7 minutes per side or until fully cooked.

5. Toast the whole wheat burger buns on the grill.

6. Assemble the burgers with lettuce, tomato slices, and a dollop of tzatziki sauce.

7. Serve the Spinach and Feta Turkey Burgers for a flavorful and healthy meal.

Nutrition:

Calories - 300 | Protein - 25g | Carbs - 25g | Fat - 12g | Fiber - 5g

Prep time: 15 minutes | Cook time: 15 minutes | Servings: 4

Mediterranean Stuffed Bell Peppers with Ground Beef

Ingredients:

- 4 bell peppers, halved and seeds removed

- 1 pound lean ground beef

- 1 cup cooked quinoa

- 1 cup cherry tomatoes, diced

- 1/2 cup red onion, finely chopped

- 1/4 cup Kalamata olives, chopped

- 2 cloves garlic, minced

- 1 teaspoon dried oregano

- 1 teaspoon dried basil

- Salt and black pepper to taste

- 1/4 cup crumbled feta cheese (optional)

- Fresh parsley for garnish

Instructions:
1. Preheat the oven to 375°F (190°C).

2. In a large skillet, brown the ground beef over medium heat until fully cooked. Drain excess fat.

3. In a large mixing bowl, combine cooked ground beef, cooked quinoa, cherry tomatoes, red onion, Kalamata olives, minced garlic, dried oregano, dried basil, salt, and black pepper.

4. Stuff each bell pepper half with the beef and quinoa mixture, pressing down gently.

5. Place the stuffed peppers in a baking dish, cover with aluminum foil, and bake for 25-30 minutes or until the peppers are tender.

6. If using, sprinkle crumbled feta cheese over the stuffed peppers during the last 5 minutes of baking.

7. Garnish with fresh parsley before serving.

8. Serve the Mediterranean Stuffed Bell Peppers with a side salad for a complete and nutritious meal.

Nutrition:
Calories - 350 | Protein - 25g | Carbs - 30g | Fat - 15g | Fiber - 7g

Prep time: 20 minutes | Cook time:30 minutes | Servings: 4

Garlic and Herb Marinated Pork Tenderloin

Ingredients:
- 1 pork tenderloin (about 1 pound)

- 4 cloves garlic, minced

- 2 tablespoons olive oil

- 1 tablespoon fresh rosemary, finely chopped

- 1 tablespoon fresh thyme, finely chopped

- 1 teaspoon dried oregano

- Zest of one lemon

- Juice of half a lemon

- Salt and black pepper to taste

Instructions:
1. Preheat the oven to 400°F (200°C).

2. In a small bowl, combine minced garlic, olive oil, rosemary, thyme, dried oregano, lemon zest, and lemon juice.

3. Season the pork tenderloin with salt and black pepper.

4. Place the pork tenderloin in a resealable plastic bag or a shallow dish. Pour the garlic and herb marinade over the pork, ensuring it's well-coated. Marinate for at least 30 minutes, or refrigerate overnight for more flavor.

5. Heat a skillet over medium-high heat. Sear the pork tenderloin on all sides until browned.

6. Transfer the pork to a baking dish and roast in the preheated oven for 20-25 minutes or until the internal temperature reaches 145°F (63°C).

7. Let the pork rest for 5 minutes before slicing.

8. Serve the Garlic and Herb Marinated Pork Tenderloin with your favorite roasted vegetables or a side salad.

Nutrition:
Calories - 250 | Protein - 30g | Carbs - 2g | Fat - 13g | Fiber - 1g

Prep time: 10 minutes (+marinating time) | Cook time: 25 minutes | Servings: 3-4

Herb-Crusted Lamb Chops with Mint Yogurt Sauce

Ingredients:
- 8 lamb chops

- 2 tablespoons fresh rosemary, finely chopped

- 2 tablespoons fresh thyme, finely chopped

- 2 cloves garlic, minced

- 2 tablespoons olive oil

- Salt and black pepper to taste

Mint Yogurt Sauce:

- 1/2 cup Greek yogurt

- 2 tablespoons fresh mint, finely chopped

- 1 tablespoon lemon juice

- Salt and black pepper to taste

Instructions:

1. Preheat the oven to 400°F (200°C).

2. In a small bowl, combine chopped rosemary, thyme, minced garlic, olive oil, salt, and black pepper to create the herb crust.

3. Rub the herb crust mixture over each lamb chop, ensuring they are evenly coated.

4. Heat an oven-safe skillet over medium-high heat. Sear the lamb chops on each side for 2-3 minutes until golden brown.

5. Transfer the skillet to the preheated oven and roast the lamb chops for 10-12 minutes for medium-rare or longer if desired.

6. While cooking lamb chops, prepare the mint yogurt sauce by combining Greek yogurt, chopped mint, lemon juice, salt, and black pepper in a bowl. Mix well.

7. Once the lamb chops are cooked to your liking, remove them from the oven and let them rest for a few minutes.

8. Serve the Herb-Crusted Lamb Chops with a dollop of Mint Yogurt Sauce on the side.

Nutrition:

Calories - 350 | Protein - 30g | Carbs - 2g | Fat - 24g | Fiber - 1g

Prep time: 15 minutes | Cook time: 15 minutes | Servings: 4

Spicy Grilled Chicken Fajitas

Ingredients:

- 1 pound boneless, skinless chicken breasts, thinly sliced

- 1 red bell pepper, thinly sliced

- 1 green bell pepper, thinly sliced

- 1 yellow onion, thinly sliced

- 2 tablespoons olive oil

- 2 tablespoons lime juice

- 2 teaspoons chili powder

- 1 teaspoon cumin

- 1 teaspoon smoked paprika

- 1/2 teaspoon cayenne pepper (adjust to taste)

- Salt and black pepper to taste

- 8 whole wheat or corn tortillas

Optional toppings:

- Salsa

- Guacamole

- Greek yogurt or sour cream

- Fresh cilantro, chopped

Instructions:
1. In a bowl, combine olive oil, lime juice, chili powder, cumin, smoked paprika, cayenne pepper, salt, and black pepper to create the marinade.

2. Place sliced chicken in the marinade, ensuring it's well-coated. Marinate for at least 30 minutes, or refrigerate for up to 4 hours for more flavor.

3. Preheat the grill or grill pan over medium-high heat.

4. In a large skillet over medium heat, sauté sliced bell peppers and onions until softened and slightly caramelized.

5. Grill the marinated chicken slices for 4-5 minutes per side or until fully cooked.

6. Warm the tortillas on the grill or in a dry skillet for about 20 seconds on each side.

7. Assemble the fajitas by placing grilled chicken, sautéed bell peppers, and onions on each tortilla.

8. Serve the Spicy Grilled Chicken Fajitas with your choice of toppings.

Nutrition:
Calories - 300 | Protein - 25g | Carbs - 30g | Fat - 10g | Fiber - 5g

Ginger Soy Glazed Beef Stir-Fry

Ingredients:
- 1 pound flank steak, thinly sliced

- 2 tablespoons soy sauce

- 1 tablespoon oyster sauce

- 1 tablespoon hoisin sauce

- 1 tablespoon rice vinegar

- 1 tablespoon honey

- 1 tablespoon fresh ginger, grated

- 2 cloves garlic, minced

- 2 tablespoons vegetable oil

- 1 red bell pepper, thinly sliced

- 1 yellow bell pepper, thinly sliced

- 1 cup broccoli florets

- 2 green onions, sliced

- Sesame seeds for garnish

- Cooked brown rice for serving

Instructions:
1. Mix soy sauce, oyster sauce, hoisin sauce, rice vinegar, honey, grated ginger, and minced garlic to create the glaze.

2. Place sliced flank steak in a separate bowl and pour half of the glaze over it. Let it marinate for at least 15 minutes.

3. Heat vegetable oil in a wok or large skillet over high heat.

4. Add marinated beef to the hot wok and stir-fry for 2-3 minutes until browned and cooked to your liking. Remove the beef from the wok and set aside.

5. In the same wok, stir-fry sliced bell peppers and broccoli until they are crisp-tender.

6. Add the cooked beef back to the wok and pour the remaining glaze over the mixture. Toss everything together until well coated and heated through.

7. Sprinkle sliced green onions and sesame seeds over the stir-fry for garnish.

8. Serve the Ginger Soy Glazed Beef Stir-Fry over cooked brown rice.

Nutrition:
Calories - 400 | Protein - 30g | Carbs - 25g | Fat - 20g | Fiber - 4g

Prep time: 20 minutes (+marinating time) | Cook time: 15 minutes | Servings: 4

Cranberry Balsamic Glazed Chicken Drumsticks

Ingredients:
- 2 pounds chicken drumsticks

- 1/2 cup cranberry sauce

- 2 tablespoons balsamic vinegar

- 1 tablespoon soy sauce

- 1 tablespoon honey

- 1 teaspoon Dijon mustard

- 2 cloves garlic, minced

- Salt and black pepper to taste

- Fresh parsley for garnish

Instructions:
1. Preheat the oven to 400°F (200°C).

2. Combine cranberry sauce, balsamic vinegar, soy sauce, honey, Dijon mustard, minced garlic, salt, and black pepper in a saucepan. Heat over medium heat, stirring, until the cranberry sauce is melted and the ingredients are well combined.

3. Place chicken drumsticks in a baking dish and pour half of the cranberry balsamic glaze over them, ensuring they are well-coated.

4. Bake in the preheated oven for 25-30 minutes, turning the drumsticks halfway through and basting them with the remaining glaze.

5. Remove from the oven Once the chicken is cooked and the glaze is caramelized.

6. Garnish with fresh parsley before serving.

7. Serve the Cranberry Balsamic Glazed Chicken Drumsticks with your favorite side dishes.

Nutrition:
Calories - 300 | Protein - 25g | Carbs - 15g | Fat - 15g | Fiber - 1g

Prep time: 15 minutes | Cook time: 30 minutes | Servings: 4-6

Dijon Mustard and Honey Glazed Pork Chops

Ingredients:
- 4 bone-in pork chops

- 3 tablespoons Dijon mustard

- 2 tablespoons honey

- 1 tablespoon olive oil

- 2 cloves garlic, minced

- 1 teaspoon dried thyme

- Salt and black pepper to taste

- Fresh parsley for garnish

Instructions:
1. Preheat the oven to 375°F (190°C).

2. Whisk together Dijon mustard, honey, olive oil, minced garlic, dried thyme, salt, and black pepper to create the glaze.

3. Season the pork chops with additional salt and black pepper.

4. Heat a skillet over medium-high heat. Sear the pork chops on each side for 2-3 minutes until golden brown.

5. Transfer the pork chops to a baking dish and brush them generously with the Dijon mustard and honey glaze.

6. Bake in the preheated oven for 20-25 minutes or until the internal temperature reaches 145°F (63°C).

7. During the last 5 minutes of baking, broil the pork chops for a caramelized finish.

8. Garnish with fresh parsley before serving.

9. Serve the Dijon Mustard and Honey Glazed Pork Chops with your favorite roasted vegetables or a side salad.

Prep time: 15 minutes | Cook time: 25 minutes | Servings: 4

Herbed Grilled Lamb Skewers

Ingredients:
- 1 pound lamb, cut into cubes

- 2 tablespoons olive oil

- 2 tablespoons fresh mint, chopped

- 2 tablespoons fresh rosemary, chopped

- 2 cloves garlic, minced

- 1 tablespoon lemon juice

- Salt and black pepper to taste

Mint Yogurt Dipping Sauce:

- 1/2 cup Greek yogurt

- 2 tablespoons fresh mint, chopped

- 1 tablespoon lemon juice

- Salt and black pepper to taste

Instructions:
1. In a bowl, combine olive oil, chopped mint, chopped rosemary, minced garlic, lemon juice, salt, and black pepper to create the marinade.

2. Place lamb cubes in the marinade, ensuring they are well-coated. Marinate for at least 30 minutes, or refrigerate for up to 4 hours for enhanced flavor.

3. Preheat the grill or grill pan over medium-high heat.

4. Thread marinated lamb cubes onto skewers.

5. Grill the lamb skewers for 8-10 minutes, turning occasionally, until they are cooked to your liking.

6. While the lamb is grilling, prepare the mint yogurt dipping sauce by combining Greek yogurt, chopped mint, lemon juice, salt, and black pepper in a bowl. Mix well.

7. Serve the Herbed Grilled Lamb Skewers with the Mint Yogurt Dipping Sauce on the side.

Nutrition:
Calories - 300 | Protein - 25g | Carbs - 2g | Fat - 20g | Fiber - 1g

Prep time: 20 minutes (+marinating time) | Cook time: 10 minutes | Servings: 4

Chipotle Lime Grilled Chicken Wings

Ingredients:
- 2 pounds chicken wings, split at joints, tips discarded

- 2 tablespoons olive oil

- 2 tablespoons lime juice

- 1 tablespoon chipotle chili powder

- 1 teaspoon ground cumin

- 1 teaspoon smoked paprika

- 2 cloves garlic, minced

- Salt and black pepper to taste

- Fresh cilantro for garnish

- Lime wedges for serving

Instructions:
1. Whisk together olive oil, lime juice, chipotle chili powder, ground cumin, smoked paprika, minced garlic, salt, and black pepper to create the marinade.

2. Place chicken wings in the marinade, ensuring they are well-coated. Marinate for at least 30 minutes, or refrigerate for up to 4 hours for a more intense flavor.

3. Preheat the grill to medium-high heat.

4. Remove the chicken wings from the marinade and let the excess drip off.

5. Grill the chicken wings for 20-25 minutes, turning occasionally until golden brown and cooked through.

6. Garnish with fresh cilantro before serving.

7. Serve the Chipotle Lime Grilled Chicken Wings with lime wedges on the side.

Nutrition:
Calories - 350 | Protein - 25g | Carbs - 2g | Fat - 28g | Fiber - 1g

Garlic Rosemary Roasted Leg of Lamb

Ingredients:
- 1 leg of lamb (approximately 5 pounds)

- 4 cloves garlic, minced

- 2 tablespoons fresh rosemary, chopped

- 2 tablespoons olive oil

- Salt and black pepper to taste

- 1 cup red wine (for basting, optional)

Instructions:
1. Preheat the oven to 375°F (190°C).

2. In a small bowl, combine minced garlic, chopped rosemary, olive oil, salt, and black pepper to create the marinade.

3. Score the surface of the leg of the lamb with a sharp knife.

4. Rub the marinade all over the leg of the lamb, ensuring it gets into the cuts.

5. Place the leg of lamb in a roasting pan.

6. Roast in the preheated oven for 1.5 to 2 hours or until the internal temperature reaches your desired doneness (140°F/60°C for medium-rare, 160°F/71°C for medium).

7. Baste the lamb with red wine (if using) every 30 minutes for added flavor and moisture.

8. Let the roasted leg of lamb rest for 15 minutes before carving.

9. Serve the Garlic Rosemary Roasted Leg of Lamb as the centerpiece of your meal.

Nutrition:
Calories - 300 | Protein - 30g | Carbs - 0g | Fat - 20g | Fiber - 0g

Prep time: 15 minutes | Cook time: 1.5-2 hours | Servings: 6-8

Barbecue Chicken and Quinoa Stuffed Bell Peppers

Ingredients:
- 4 bell peppers, halved and seeds removed

- 1 cup cooked quinoa

- 1 cup shredded cooked chicken

- 1/2 cup black beans, drained and rinsed

- 1/2 cup corn kernels

- 1/2 cup barbecue sauce

- 1/2 cup shredded cheddar cheese

- 2 green onions, sliced

- Fresh cilantro for garnish

Instructions:
1. Preheat the oven to 375°F (190°C).

2. combine cooked quinoa, shredded chicken, black beans, corn, and barbecue sauce in a bowl.

3. Spoon the quinoa mixture into halved bell peppers, pressing down gently.

4. Top each stuffed pepper with shredded cheddar cheese.

5. Place the stuffed peppers in a baking dish.

6. Bake in the preheated oven for 25-30 minutes or until the peppers are tender.

7. Garnish with sliced green onions and fresh cilantro before serving.

8. Serve the Barbecue Chicken and Quinoa Stuffed Bell Peppers as a wholesome meal.

Nutrition:
Calories - 350 | Protein - 20g | Carbs - 40g | Fat - 15g | Fiber - 6g

Prep time: 20 minutes | Cook time: 25-30 minutes | Servings: 4

Italian Herb Marinated Grilled Pork Chops

Ingredients:
- 4 bone-in pork chops

- 1/4 cup olive oil

- 2 tablespoons balsamic vinegar

- 1 tablespoon Italian seasoning

- 1 teaspoon garlic powder

- Salt and black pepper to taste

- Fresh basil for garnish

Instructions:
1. In a bowl, whisk together olive oil, balsamic vinegar, Italian seasoning, garlic powder, salt, and black pepper to create the marinade.

2. Place pork chops in the marinade, ensuring they are well-coated. Marinate for at least 30 minutes.

3. Preheat the grill to medium-high heat.

4. Grill the marinated pork chops for 4-5 minutes per side or until fully cooked.

5. Garnish with fresh basil before serving.

6. Serve the Italian Herb Marinated Grilled Pork Chops with your favorite side dishes.

Nutrition:
Calories - 350 | Protein - 30g | Carbs - 2g | Fat - 25g | Fiber - 0g

Prep time: 15 minutes (+marinating time) | Cook time: 10 minutes | Servings: 4

Apple Cider Vinegar Marinated Grilled Pork Tenderloin

Ingredients:
- 1 pork tenderloin (approximately 1 pound)

- 1/4 cup apple cider vinegar

- 2 tablespoons olive oil

- 1 tablespoon Dijon mustard

- 1 tablespoon honey

- 2 cloves garlic, minced

- 1 teaspoon dried thyme

- Salt and black pepper to taste

- Fresh parsley for garnish

Instructions:

1. Whisk together apple cider vinegar, olive oil, Dijon mustard, honey, minced garlic, dried thyme, salt, and black pepper to create the marinade.

2. Place the pork tenderloin in a resealable plastic bag and pour the marinade over it. Seal the bag and marinate in the refrigerator for at least 2 hours or overnight for maximum flavor.

3. Preheat the grill to medium-high heat.

4. Remove the pork tenderloin from the marinade and discard the marinade.

5. Grill the pork tenderloin for 15-20 minutes, turning occasionally, until it reaches an internal temperature of 145°F (63°C).

6. Let the grilled pork tenderloin rest for 5 minutes before slicing.

7. Garnish with fresh parsley before serving.

8. Serve the Apple Cider Vinegar Marinated Grilled Pork Tenderloin with your favorite sides.

Nutrition:
Calories - 250 | Protein - 25g | Carbs - 5g | Fat - 15g | Fiber - 0g

Prep time: 15 minutes (+marinating time) | Cook time: 20 minutes | Servings: 3-4

Lemon Pepper Baked Chicken Thighs

Ingredients:
- 8 chicken thighs, bone-in, skin-on

- 2 tablespoons olive oil

- Zest and juice of 1 lemon

- 1 tablespoon dried oregano

- 1 tablespoon garlic powder

- 1 teaspoon onion powder

- 1 teaspoon black pepper

- Salt to taste

- Fresh parsley for garnish

Instructions:
1. Preheat the oven to 400°F (200°C).

2. Mix olive oil, lemon zest, lemon juice, dried oregano, garlic powder, onion powder, black pepper, and salt in a bowl.

3. Place chicken thighs in a baking dish and brush them with the lemon-pepper mixture, ensuring they are well-coated.

4. Bake in the preheated oven for 30-35 minutes or until the chicken thighs are golden brown and cooked through.

5. Garnish with fresh parsley before serving.

6. Serve the Lemon Pepper Baked Chicken Thighs with your favorite roasted vegetables or salad.

Nutrition:
Calories - 350 | Protein - 25g | Carbs - 2g | Fat - 28g | Fiber - 1g

Prep time: 15 minutes | Cook time: 30-35 minutes | Servings: 4

Pineapple Teriyaki Beef Skewers

Ingredients:
- 1 pound beef sirloin, cut into cubes

- 1 cup pineapple chunks

- 1/4 cup soy sauce

- 2 tablespoons pineapple juice

- 2 tablespoons honey

- 1 tablespoon rice vinegar

- 1 teaspoon sesame oil

- 2 cloves garlic, minced

- 1 teaspoon grated ginger

- Wooden skewers, soaked in water

Instructions:
1. Whisk together soy sauce, pineapple juice, honey, rice vinegar, sesame oil, minced garlic, and grated ginger to create the teriyaki marinade.

2. Thread beef cubes and pineapple chunks onto the soaked wooden skewers.

3. Place the skewers in a shallow dish and pour the teriyaki marinade over them. Marinate for at least 30 minutes.

4. Preheat the grill to medium-high heat.

5. Grill the beef skewers for 8-10 minutes, turning occasionally, until the beef is cooked to your liking.

6. Serve the Pineapple Teriyaki Beef Skewers over cooked brown rice or quinoa.

Nutrition:
Calories - 300 | Protein - 25g | Carbs - 15g | Fat - 15g | Fiber - 2g

Prep time: 20 minutes (+marinating time) | Cook time: 10 minutes | Servings: 4-6

Greek-Style Stuffed Bell Peppers with Ground Lamb

Ingredients:
- 4 bell peppers, halved and seeds removed

- 1 pound ground lamb

- 1 cup cooked quinoa

- 1 cup cherry tomatoes, halved

- 1/2 cup feta cheese, crumbled

- 1/4 cup Kalamata olives, chopped

- 1/4 cup red onion, finely chopped

- 2 cloves garlic, minced

- 1 teaspoon dried oregano

- 1 teaspoon dried basil

- Salt and black pepper to taste

- Fresh parsley for garnish

Instructions:
1. Preheat the oven to 375°F (190°C).

2. Brown the ground lamb until fully cooked in a skillet over medium heat. Drain excess fat.

3. Combine cooked quinoa, browned lamb, cherry tomatoes, feta cheese, Kalamata olives, red onion, minced garlic, dried oregano, dried basil, salt, and black pepper in a large bowl.

4. Stuff each bell pepper half with the lamb and quinoa mixture.

5. Place the stuffed peppers in a baking dish.

6. Bake in the preheated oven for 25-30 minutes or until the peppers are tender.

7. Garnish with fresh parsley before serving.

8. Serve the Greek-style stuffed Bell Peppers with a side of tzatziki sauce.

Nutrition:
Calories - 350 | Protein - 20g | Carbs - 25g | Fat - 18g | Fiber - 5g

Prep time: 20 minutes | Cook time: 25-30 minutes | Servings: 4

Honey Mustard Glazed Chicken Breasts

Ingredients:
- 4 boneless, skinless chicken breasts

- 1/4 cup Dijon mustard

- 2 tablespoons honey

- 1 tablespoon whole-grain mustard

- 1 tablespoon olive oil

- 2 cloves garlic, minced

- 1 teaspoon dried thyme

- Salt and black pepper to taste

- Fresh chives for garnish

Instructions:
1. Preheat the oven to 400°F (200°C).

2. Mix Dijon mustard, honey, whole grain mustard, olive oil, minced garlic, dried thyme, salt, and black pepper in a bowl.

3. Place chicken breasts in a baking dish and brush them with the honey mustard glaze, ensuring they are well-coated.

4. Bake in the preheated oven for 20-25 minutes or until the chicken is cooked through.

5. Garnish with fresh chives before serving.

6. Serve the Honey Mustard Glazed Chicken Breasts with steamed vegetables or a side salad.

Nutrition:
Calories - 300 | Protein - 30g | Carbs - 15g | Fat - 12g | Fiber - 1g

Prep time: 15 minutes | Cook time: 20-25 minutes | Servings: 4

Spiced Orange Glazed Pork Loin

Ingredients:
- 1 pork loin (approximately 2 pounds)

- Zest and juice of 1 orange

- 1/4 cup soy sauce

- 2 tablespoons honey

- 1 tablespoon olive oil

- 1 teaspoon ground ginger

- 1 teaspoon ground cinnamon

- 1/2 teaspoon ground cloves

- Salt and black pepper to taste

- Orange slices for garnish

Instructions:
1. Preheat the oven to 375°F (190°C).

2. Mix together orange zest, orange juice, soy sauce, honey, olive oil, ground ginger, cinnamon, cloves, salt, and black pepper to create the spiced orange glaze.

3. Place the pork loin in a roasting pan and brush it with the spiced orange glaze, ensuring it is well-coated.

4. Roast in the preheated oven for 1 to 1.5 hours or until the internal temperature reaches 145°F (63°C).

5. Baste the pork loin with the glaze every 20-30 minutes for added flavor.

6. Let the roasted pork loin rest for 10 minutes before slicing.

7. Garnish with orange slices before serving.

8. Serve the Spiced Orange Glazed Pork Loin with roasted vegetables or quinoa.

Nutrition:
Calories - 350 | Protein - 30g | Carbs - 15g | Fat - 18g | Fiber - 2g

Prep time: 20 minutes | Cook time: 1-1.5 hours | Servings: 6-8

Slow-Cooked Pulled Pork Tacos

Ingredients:
- 3 pounds pork shoulder, trimmed

- 1 large onion, sliced

- 4 cloves garlic, minced

- 1 cup chicken broth

- 1/2 cup barbecue sauce

- 2 tablespoons apple cider vinegar

- 1 tablespoon brown sugar

- 1 tablespoon smoked paprika

- 1 teaspoon cumin

- 1 teaspoon chili powder

- Salt and black pepper to taste

- Corn tortillas

- Coleslaw for topping

- Fresh cilantro for garnish

Instructions:
1. Place the sliced onion and minced garlic at the bottom of the slow cooker.

2. Season the pork shoulder with salt, black pepper, smoked paprika, cumin, and chili powder.

3. Place the seasoned pork shoulder on top of the onions and garlic in the slow cooker.

4. Mix chicken broth, barbecue sauce, apple cider vinegar, and brown sugar in a bowl. Pour the mixture over the pork.

5. Cook on low for 8-10 hours or until the pork is tender and easily shreds.

6. Shred the pork using two forks and mix it with the cooking juices.

7. Warm the corn tortillas and fill them with the pulled pork.

8. Top with coleslaw and garnish with fresh cilantro.

9. Serve the Slow-Cooked Pulled Pork Tacos with lime wedges on the side.

Nutrition:
Calories - 400 | Protein - 25g | Carbs - 25g | Fat - 20g | Fiber - 3g

Prep time: 15 minutes | Cook time: 8-10 hours (slow cooker) | Servings: 6-8

Moroccan Spiced Lamb Kabobs

Ingredients:
- 1 pound lamb, cubed

- 1 bell pepper, cut into chunks

- 1 red onion, cut into chunks

- 1 zucchini, sliced

- 1/4 cup olive oil

- 2 tablespoons lemon juice

- 1 teaspoon ground cumin

- 1 teaspoon ground coriander

- 1 teaspoon smoked paprika

- 1/2 teaspoon cinnamon

- 1/2 teaspoon cayenne pepper

- Salt and black pepper to taste

- Fresh mint for garnish

Instructions:
1. Mix olive oil, lemon juice, ground cumin, coriander, smoked paprika, cinnamon, cayenne pepper, salt, and black pepper to create the marinade.

2. Thread lamb cubes, bell pepper, red onion, and zucchini onto skewers.

3. Brush the kabobs with the marinade, ensuring they are well-coated.

4. Preheat the grill to medium-high heat.

5. Grill the lamb kabobs for 10-12 minutes, turning occasionally, until the lamb is cooked to your liking.

6. Garnish with fresh mint before serving.

7. Serve the Moroccan Spiced Lamb Kabobs with couscous or a Mediterranean salad.

Nutrition:
Calories - 350 | Protein - 20g | Carbs - 10g | Fat - 25g | Fiber - 3g

Prep time: 20 minutes (+marinating time) | Cook time: 10-12 minutes | Servings: 4

Tuscan Herb Roasted Chicken Thighs

Ingredients:
- 8 chicken thighs, bone-in, skin-on

- 1/4 cup olive oil

- 2 tablespoons balsamic vinegar

- 1 tablespoon dried rosemary

- 1 tablespoon dried thyme

- 1 tablespoon dried oregano

- 4 cloves garlic, minced

- Salt and black pepper to taste

- Lemon wedges for serving

- Fresh parsley for garnish

Instructions:
1. Preheat the oven to 425°F (220°C).

2. Mix in a bowl in olive oil, balsamic vinegar, rosemary, thyme, oregano, minced garlic, salt, and black pepper.

3. Place chicken thighs in a baking dish and brush them with the herb-infused olive oil mixture, ensuring they are well-coated.

4. Roast in the preheated oven for 30-35 minutes or until the chicken thighs are golden brown and cooked through.

5. Garnish with fresh parsley and serve with lemon wedges.

Nutrition
Calories - 400 | Protein - 30g | Carbs - 2g | Fat - 30g | Fiber - 0g

Citrus Glazed Chicken Skewers

Ingredients:
- 1.5 pounds boneless, skinless chicken breasts cut into chunks

- 1/4 cup orange juice

- 2 tablespoons lemon juice

- 2 tablespoons lime juice

- 1/4 cup honey

- 2 tablespoons soy sauce

- 1 tablespoon olive oil

- 2 cloves garlic, minced

- 1 teaspoon dried thyme

- Salt and black pepper to taste

- Wooden skewers soaked in water

- Orange, lemon, and lime slices for garnish

Instructions:
1. Mix orange juice, lemon juice, lime juice, honey, soy sauce, olive oil, minced garlic, dried thyme, salt, and black pepper to create the citrus glaze.

2. Thread chicken chunks onto soaked wooden skewers.

3. Brush the chicken skewers with the citrus glaze, ensuring they are well-coated.

4. Preheat the grill to medium-high heat.

5. Grill the chicken skewers for 10-12 minutes, turning occasionally, until cooked through.

6. Garnish with orange, lemon, and lime slices before serving.

7. Serve the Citrus Glazed Chicken Skewers with a side of quinoa or a green salad.

Nutrition:
Calories - 300 | Protein - 25g | Carbs - 20g | Fat - 12g | Fiber - 1g

Prep time: 15 minutes (+marinating time) | Cook time: 10-12 minutes | Servings: 4

Cumin-Spiced Turkey Burgers with Avocado

Ingredients:
- 1.5 pounds ground turkey

- 1/4 cup breadcrumbs

- 1/4 cup red onion, finely chopped

- 2 tablespoons ground cumin

- 1 teaspoon smoked paprika

- 1 teaspoon garlic powder

- Salt and black pepper to taste

- Whole-grain burger buns

- Avocado slices for topping

- Fresh lettuce and tomato slices for garnish

Instructions:
1. Combine ground turkey, breadcrumbs, chopped red onion, ground cumin, smoked paprika, garlic powder, salt, and black pepper in a bowl. Mix until well combined.

2. Divide the mixture into equal portions and shape them into burger patties.

3. Preheat the grill or stovetop grill pan to medium-high heat.

4. Grill the turkey burgers for 5-6 minutes per side or until cooked through.

5. Toast the whole-grain burger buns on the grill.

6. Assemble the burgers with avocado slices, fresh lettuce, and tomato slices.

7. Serve the Cumin-Spiced Turkey Burgers with a side of sweet potato fries or a green salad.

Nutrition:
Calories - 350 | Protein - 30g | Carbs - 25g | Fat - 15g | Fiber - 5g

Prep time: 20 minutes | Cook time: 10-12 minutes | Servings: 4

Basil Pesto Chicken with Roasted Vegetables

Ingredients:
- 4 boneless, skinless chicken breasts

- 1 cup cherry tomatoes, halved

- 1 zucchini, sliced

- 1 red bell pepper, sliced

- 1/4 cup basil pesto

- 2 tablespoons olive oil

- 2 cloves garlic, minced

- Salt and black pepper to taste

- Fresh basil for garnish

Instructions:
1. Preheat the oven to 400°F (200°C).

2. Place chicken breasts in a baking dish.

3. Mix cherry tomatoes, sliced zucchini, sliced red bell pepper, basil pesto, olive oil, minced garlic, salt, and black pepper in a bowl.

4. Spoon the vegetable mixture over the chicken breasts.

5. Roast in the preheated oven for 25-30 minutes or until the chicken is cooked through.

6. Garnish with fresh basil before serving.

7. Serve the Basil Pesto Chicken with Roasted Vegetables over quinoa or brown rice.

Nutrition:
Calories - 350 | Protein - 30g | Carbs - 10g | Fat - 20g | Fiber - 3g

Prep time: 15 minutes | Cook time: 25-30 minutes | Servings: 4

Grilled Lemon Herb Chicken Breasts

Ingredients:
- 4 boneless, skinless chicken breasts

- 1/4 cup olive oil

- Zest and juice of 1 lemon

- 2 tablespoons fresh parsley, chopped

- 1 tablespoon fresh thyme, chopped

- 1 tablespoon fresh rosemary, chopped

- 2 cloves garlic, minced

- Salt and black pepper to taste

- Lemon slices for garnish

Instructions:
1. Whisk together olive oil, lemon zest, lemon juice, chopped parsley, chopped thyme, chopped rosemary, minced garlic, salt, and black pepper to create the marinade.

2. Place the chicken breasts in a shallow dish and pour the marinade over them. Ensure the chicken is well-coated.

3. Marinate in the refrigerator for at least 30 minutes, or preferably overnight.

4. Preheat the grill to medium-high heat.

5. Grill the chicken breasts for 6-8 minutes per side or until cooked through.

6. Garnish with lemon slices before serving.

7. Serve the Grilled Lemon Herb Chicken Breasts with a side of quinoa or grilled vegetables.

Nutrition
 Calories - 300 | Protein - 25g | Carbs - 2g | Fat - 20g | Fiber - 1g

Prep time: 15 minutes (+marinating time) | Cook time: 12-16 minutes | Servings: 4

Rosemary Balsamic Roasted Turkey

Ingredients:
- 1 whole turkey (12-14 pounds), thawed

- 1/2 cup olive oil

- 1/4 cup balsamic vinegar

- 2 tablespoons fresh rosemary, chopped

- 2 tablespoons Dijon mustard

- 4 cloves garlic, minced

- Salt and black pepper to taste

- Fresh rosemary sprigs for garnish

- Cranberry sauce for serving

Instructions:
1. Preheat the oven to 325°F (165°C).

2. Whisk together olive oil, balsamic vinegar, chopped rosemary, Dijon mustard, minced garlic, salt, and black pepper to create the marinade.

3. Place the turkey in a roasting pan.

4. Brush the turkey with the rosemary balsamic marinade, ensuring it is well-coated.

5. Roast in the preheated oven, basting every 30 minutes, until the internal temperature reaches 165°F (74°C).

6. Let the turkey rest for 20 minutes before carving.

7. Garnish with fresh rosemary sprigs.

8. Serve the Rosemary Balsamic Roasted Turkey with cranberry sauce and your favorite sides.

Nutrition:
Calories - 350 | Protein - 30g | Carbs - 2g | Fat - 25g | Fiber - 0g

Prep time: 20 minutes (+marinating time) | Cook time: Varies based on turkey size | Servings: 8-10

Cranberry-Orange Glazed Veal

Ingredients:
- 500g veal slices

- 1/2 cup cranberry juice (120ml)

- Juice of 2 oranges

- 2 tbsp soy sauce

- 2 tbsp honey

- 2 tsp cornstarch

- 2 tbsp vegetable oil

- 2 cloves garlic, minced

- Salt and pepper to taste

- Green onions and cilantro for garnish

Instructions:
1. Heat vegetable oil in a deep skillet.

2. Sear veal slices until golden brown.

3. Mix cranberry juice, orange juice, soy sauce, honey, and cornstarch in a bowl.

4. Add the mixture to the skillet with the meat, stirring until the sauce thickens.

5. Season with salt and pepper, add minced garlic.

6. Cook on medium heat until the sauce becomes thick and glossy.

7. Serve Cranberry-Orange Glazed Veal, garnished with chopped green onions and cilantro.

8. Pair with mashed potatoes or steamed rice.

Nutrition:
Calories - 300 | Protein - 25g | Carbs - 15g | Fat - 15g | Fiber - 2g

Prep time: 20 minutes | Servings: 4

Lamb Patties with Cilantro and Spices

Ingredients:
- 500g ground lamb

- 1/2 cup breadcrumbs

- 1/4 cup fresh cilantro, chopped

- 2 cloves garlic, minced

- 1 tsp ground cumin

- 1 tsp ground coriander

- 1/2 tsp paprika

- Salt and pepper to taste

- 2 tbsp olive oil

- Fresh cilantro leaves for garnish

Instructions:

1. Combine ground lamb, breadcrumbs, chopped cilantro, minced garlic, cumin, coriander, paprika, salt, and pepper in a bowl. Mix until well combined.

2. Shape the mixture into patties.

3. Heat olive oil in a skillet over medium-high heat.

4. Cook the lamb patties for 4-5 minutes per side or until they reach your desired level of doneness.

5. Garnish with fresh cilantro leaves before serving.

6. Serve the Lamb Patties with Cilantro and Spices with a side of couscous or roasted vegetables.

Nutrition:
Calories - 350 | Protein - 25g | Carbs - 10g | Fat - 22g | Fiber - 2g

Prep time: 15 minutes | Cook time: 10-12 minutes | Servings: 4

Dijon and Honey Glazed Tilapia

Ingredients:
- 4 tilapia fillets

- 2 tablespoons Dijon mustard

- 1 tablespoon honey

- 1 tablespoon olive oil

- 2 cloves garlic, minced

- 1 teaspoon dried thyme

- Salt and black pepper to taste

- Lemon wedges for serving

- Fresh parsley for garnish

Instructions:
1. Preheat the oven to 375°F (190°C).

2. Whisk together Dijon mustard, honey, olive oil, minced garlic, dried thyme, salt, and black pepper in a small bowl.

3. Place tilapia fillets on a baking sheet lined with parchment paper.

4. Brush the Dijon and honey glaze over each fillet, ensuring they are well-coated.

5. Bake in the preheated oven for 12-15 minutes or until the fish flakes easily with a fork.

6. Garnish with fresh parsley and serve with lemon wedges.

Nutrition:
Calories - 180 | Protein - 25g | Carbs - 5g | Fat - 7g | Fiber - 0.5g

Prep time: 10 minutes | Cook time: 15 minutes | Servings: 4

Citrus-Infused Mahi Mahi

Ingredients:
- 4 mahi mahi fillets

- Zest and juice of 1 orange

- Zest and juice of 1 lemon

- 2 tablespoons olive oil

- 2 cloves garlic, minced

- 1 teaspoon dried oregano

- Salt and black pepper to taste

- Fresh cilantro for garnish

Instructions:
1. Mix the orange zest, orange juice, lemon zest, lemon juice, olive oil, minced garlic, dried oregano, salt, and black pepper in a bowl.

2. Place mahi mahi fillets in a shallow dish and pour the citrus-infused marinade over them. Let it marinate for at least 30 minutes.

3. Preheat the grill to medium-high heat.

4. Grill the mahi mahi fillets for 4-5 minutes per side or until they are cooked through and have grill marks.

5. Garnish with fresh cilantro before serving.

Nutrition:
Calories - 220 | Protein - 30g | Carbs - 3g | Fat - 10g | Fiber - 0.5g

Prep time: 15 minutes (+marinating time) | Cook time: 10 minutes | Servings: 4

Cajun Spiced Catfish Fillets

Ingredients:
- 4 catfish fillets

- 2 tablespoons Cajun seasoning

- 1 tablespoon olive oil

- 1 tablespoon lemon juice

- 1 teaspoon paprika

- 1/2 teaspoon garlic powder

- Salt and black pepper to taste

- Fresh thyme for garnish

Instructions:
1. Preheat the oven to 400°F (200°C).

2. In a small bowl, combine Cajun seasoning, olive oil, lemon juice, paprika, garlic powder, salt, and black pepper.

3. Rub the Cajun spice mixture over each catfish fillet.

4. Place the fillets on a baking sheet lined with parchment paper.

5. Bake in the preheated oven for 15-18 minutes or until the fish is flaky and cooked through.

6. Garnish with fresh thyme before serving.

Nutrition:
Calories - 190 | Protein - 22g | Carbs - 2g | Fat - 10g | Fiber - 0.5g

Prep time: 10 minutes | Cook time: 15-18 minutes | Servings: 4

Sesame Soy Glazed Tuna Steaks

Ingredients:
- 4 tuna steaks

- 1/4 cup soy sauce

- 2 tablespoons sesame oil

- 1 tablespoon honey

- 1 tablespoon rice vinegar

- 1 teaspoon grated ginger

- 2 cloves garlic, minced

- 1 tablespoon sesame seeds

- Green onions for garnish

Instructions:
1. Whisk together soy sauce, sesame oil, honey, rice vinegar, grated ginger, and minced garlic in a bowl.

2. Place tuna steaks in a shallow dish and pour the sesame soy glaze over them. Marinate for at least 30 minutes.

3. Preheat the grill or grill pan to high heat.

4. Grill tuna steaks for 2-3 minutes per side for medium-rare or longer for desired doneness.

5. Sprinkle sesame seeds and green onions over the tuna steaks before serving.

Nutrition:
Calories - 250 | Protein - 30g | Carbs - 5g | Fat - 12g | Fiber - 1g

Prep time: 10 minutes (+marinating time) | Cook time: 6 minutes | Servings: 4

Coconut Lime Grilled Shrimp

Ingredients:
- 1 pound large shrimp, peeled and deveined

- 1/4 cup coconut milk

- Zest and juice of 2 limes

- 2 tablespoons olive oil

- 1 tablespoon soy sauce

- 1 teaspoon honey

- 2 cloves garlic, minced

- 1 teaspoon chili flakes (optional)

- Fresh cilantro for garnish

Instructions:
1. Combine coconut milk, zest, lime juice, olive oil, soy sauce, honey, minced garlic, and chili flakes in a bowl.

2. Add the shrimp to the coconut lime marinade and let it marinate for at least 15 minutes.

3. Preheat the grill to medium-high heat.

4. Thread the marinated shrimp onto skewers and grill for 2-3 minutes per side or until they are opaque.

5. Garnish with fresh cilantro before serving.

Nutrition:
Calories - 180 | Protein - 20g | Carbs - 3g | Fat - 10g | Fiber - 0.5g

Prep time: 15 minutes (+marinating time) | Cook time: 6 minutes | Servings: 4

Teriyaki Salmon Bowls

Ingredients:
- 4 salmon fillets

- 1/2 cup teriyaki sauce

- 2 tablespoons olive oil

- 1 tablespoon honey

- 1 teaspoon grated ginger

- 2 cups cooked brown rice

- Steamed broccoli florets

- Sliced green onions for garnish

- Sesame seeds for garnish

Instructions:
1. Preheat the oven to 400°F (200°C).

2. Mix teriyaki sauce, olive oil, honey, and grated ginger in a bowl.

3. Place salmon fillets on a baking sheet lined with parchment paper and brush them with the teriyaki mixture.

4. Bake in the preheated oven for 12-15 minutes or until the salmon is cooked through.

5. Serve the teriyaki salmon over cooked brown rice and steamed broccoli.

6. Garnish with sliced green onions and sesame seeds.

Nutrition:
Calories - 350 | Protein - 25g | Carbs - 30g | Fat - 15g | Fiber - 3g

Prep time: 10 minutes | Cook time: 15 minutes | Servings: 4

Herb Marinated Grilled Sea Bass

Ingredients:
- 4 sea bass fillets

- 2 tablespoons olive oil

- Juice of 1 lemon

- 2 cloves garlic, minced

- 1 tablespoon fresh basil, chopped

- 1 tablespoon fresh parsley, chopped

- Salt and black pepper to taste

- Lemon wedges for serving

Instructions:

1. Mix olive oil, lemon juice, minced garlic, chopped basil, chopped parsley, salt, and black pepper in a bowl.

2. Place sea bass fillets in a shallow dish and pour the herb marinade over them. Let it marinate for at least 30 minutes.

3. Preheat the grill to medium-high heat.

4. Grill the sea bass fillets for 3-4 minutes per side or until they are cooked through and have grill marks.

5. Serve Herb Marinated Grilled Sea Bass with lemon wedges.

Nutrition:

Calories - 200 | Protein - 28g | Carbs - 1g | Fat - 9g | Fiber - 0.5g

Prep time: 15 minutes (+marinating time) | Cook time: 8 minutes | Servings: 4

Lemon Garlic Butter Scallops

Ingredients:

- 1 pound scallops, patted dry

- 3 tablespoons unsalted butter

- 3 cloves garlic, minced

- Zest and juice of 1 lemon

- Salt and black pepper to taste

- Fresh parsley for garnish

Instructions:

1. Heat butter in a skillet over medium-high heat until melted.

2. Add minced garlic and cook for 1-2 minutes until fragrant.

3. Add scallops to the skillet and cook for 2-3 minutes per side until they are golden brown.

4. Season with lemon zest, lemon juice, salt, and black pepper.

5. Garnish Lemon Garlic Butter Scallops with fresh parsley before serving.

Nutrition:
Calories - 180 | Protein - 20g | Carbs - 4g | Fat - 10g | Fiber - 0.5g

Prep time: 5 minutes | Cook time: 6 minutes | Servings: 4

Chili Lime Grilled Halibut

Ingredients:
- 4 halibut fillets

- 2 tablespoons olive oil

- Zest and juice of 2 limes

- 1 teaspoon chili powder

- 1/2 teaspoon cumin

- 1/2 teaspoon paprika

- Salt and black pepper to taste

- Fresh cilantro for garnish

Instructions:
1. Mix olive oil, zest, lime juice, chili powder, cumin, paprika, salt, and black pepper in a bowl.

2. Place halibut fillets in a shallow dish and pour the chili lime marinade over them. Let it marinate for at least 30 minutes.

3. Preheat the grill to medium-high heat.

4. Grill the halibut fillets for 3-4 minutes per side or until they are cooked through and have grill marks.

5. Garnish Chili Lime Grilled Halibut with fresh cilantro before serving.

Nutrition:
Calories - 220 | Protein - 30g | Carbs - 2g | Fat - 10g | Fiber - 0.5g

Garlic Parmesan Crusted Tilapia

Ingredients:
- 4 tilapia fillets

- 1/2 cup grated Parmesan cheese

- 1/4 cup breadcrumbs

- 2 cloves garlic, minced

- 2 tablespoons fresh parsley, chopped

- 2 tablespoons olive oil

- Lemon wedges for serving

- Salt and black pepper to taste

Instructions:
1. Preheat the oven to 400°F (200°C).

2. Mix grated Parmesan cheese, breadcrumbs, minced garlic, chopped parsley, salt, and black pepper in a bowl.

3. Place tilapia fillets on a baking sheet lined with parchment paper.

4. Brush each fillet with olive oil and press the Parmesan mixture onto the top of each fillet.

5. Bake in the preheated oven for 12-15 minutes or until the tilapia is cooked through and the crust is golden brown.

6. Serve Garlic Parmesan-crusted tilapia with lemon wedges.

Nutrition:
Calories - 220 | Protein - 25g | Carbs - 5g | Fat - 10g | Fiber - 0.5g

Prep time: 10 minutes | Cook time: 15 minutes | Servings: 4

Stuffed Bell Peppers with Shrimp

Ingredients:
- 4 bell peppers, halved and seeds removed

- 1 pound large shrimp, peeled and deveined

- 1 cup cherry tomatoes, halved

- 1/2 cup feta cheese, crumbled

- 1/4 cup Kalamata olives, chopped

- 2 tablespoons olive oil

- 2 cloves garlic, minced

- 1 teaspoon dried oregano

- Salt and black pepper to taste

- Fresh parsley for garnish

Instructions:
1. Preheat the oven to 375°F (190°C).

2. Mix shrimp, cherry tomatoes, feta cheese, Kalamata olives, olive oil, minced garlic, dried oregano, salt, and black pepper in a bowl.

3. Stuff each bell pepper half with the shrimp mixture.

4. Place the stuffed bell peppers on a baking sheet lined with parchment paper.

5. Bake in the preheated oven for 20-25 minutes or until the shrimp are cooked through.

6. Garnish Mediterranean Stuffed Bell Peppers with fresh parsley before serving.

Nutrition:
Calories - 280 | Protein - 25g | Carbs - 15g | Fat - 14g | Fiber - 3g

Prep time: 20 minutes | Cook time: 25 minutes | Servings: 4

Shrimp and Broccoli Stir-Fry

Ingredients:
- 1 pound large shrimp, peeled and deveined

- 4 cups broccoli florets

- 2 tablespoons soy sauce

- 1 tablespoon oyster sauce

- 1 tablespoon hoisin sauce

- 1 tablespoon sesame oil

- 2 tablespoons vegetable oil

- 2 cloves garlic, minced

- 1 teaspoon fresh ginger, grated

- Cooked brown rice for serving

Instructions:
1. Whisk together soy sauce, oyster sauce, hoisin sauce, and sesame oil in a small bowl.

2. Heat vegetable oil in a wok or large skillet over high heat.

3. Add shrimp and stir-fry for 2-3 minutes until they start to turn pink. Remove shrimp from the wok and set aside.

4. In the same wok, add a bit more oil if needed and stir-fry broccoli for 3-4 minutes until it's crisp-tender.

5. Add minced garlic and grated ginger to the wok and stir-fry for 1 minute.

6. Return the cooked shrimp to the wok and pour the sauce over the shrimp and broccoli. Stir-fry for an additional 2 minutes.

7. Serve Shrimp and Broccoli Stir-Fry over cooked brown rice.

Nutrition:
Calories - 320 | Protein - 25g | Carbs - 20g | Fat - 15g | Fiber - 5g

Prep time: 15 minutes | Cook time: 10 minutes | Servings: 4

Smoky Paprika Grilled Octopus

Ingredients:
- 1 pound octopus, cleaned and tentacles separated

- 2 tablespoons olive oil

- 1 tablespoon smoked paprika

- 1 teaspoon garlic powder

- 1 teaspoon onion powder

- 1/2 teaspoon cayenne pepper

- Salt and black pepper to taste

- Lemon wedges for serving

- Fresh parsley for garnish

Instructions:
1. Preheat the grill to medium-high heat.

2. Mix olive oil, smoked paprika, garlic powder, onion powder, cayenne pepper, salt, and black pepper in a bowl.

3. Brush the octopus tentacles with the spice mixture.

4. Grill the octopus tentacles for 3-4 minutes per side or until they are cooked through and have grill marks.

5. Serve Smoky Paprika Grilled Octopus with lemon wedges and garnish with fresh parsley.

Nutrition:
Calories - 180 | Protein - 25g | Carbs - 2g | Fat - 8g | Fiber - 0.5g

Prep time: 10 minutes (+marinating time) | Cook time: 8 minutes | Servings: 4

Almond-Crusted Baked Catfish

Ingredients:
- 4 catfish fillets

- 1/2 cup almond flour

- 1/4 cup grated Parmesan cheese

- 1 teaspoon garlic powder

- 1 teaspoon dried thyme

- 1/2 teaspoon paprika

- 2 tablespoons olive oil

- Lemon wedges for serving

- Fresh dill for garnish

- Salt and black pepper to taste

Instructions:
1. Preheat the oven to 400°F (200°C).

2. Mix almond flour, grated Parmesan cheese, garlic powder, dried thyme, paprika, salt, and black pepper in a bowl.

3. Brush each catfish fillet with olive oil and press the almond mixture onto the top of each fillet.

4. Place catfish fillets on a baking sheet lined with parchment paper.

5. Bake in the preheated oven for 15-18 minutes or until the catfish is cooked through and the crust is golden brown.

6. Serve Almond-Crusted Baked Catfish with lemon wedges and garnish with fresh dill.

Nutrition:
Calories - 220 | Protein - 20g | Carbs - 5g | Fat - 15g | Fiber - 2g

Prep time: 10 minutes | Cook time: 18 minutes | Servings: 4

Teriyaki Glazed Pineapple Salmon

Ingredients:
- 4 salmon fillets

- 1/4 cup low-sodium soy sauce

- 2 tablespoons honey

- 1 tablespoon rice vinegar

- 1 teaspoon grated ginger

- 1 clove garlic, minced

- 1/2 cup pineapple juice

- 1 cup pineapple chunks

- Green onions for garnish

- Sesame seeds for garnish

- Cooked quinoa for serving

Instructions:
1. whisk together soy sauce, honey, rice vinegar, grated ginger, minced garlic, and pineapple juice in a bowl to make the teriyaki sauce.

2. Marinate salmon fillets in the teriyaki sauce for at least 30 minutes.

3. Preheat the grill to medium-high heat.

4. Grill the salmon fillets for 4-5 minutes per side or until they are cooked through.

5. Add pineapple chunks to the grill at the last minute of grilling.

6. Serve Teriyaki Glazed Pineapple Salmon over cooked quinoa, garnished with green onions and sesame seeds.

Nutrition:
Calories - 320 | Protein - 25g | Carbs - 25g | Fat - 14g | Fiber - 3g

Prep time 15 minutes (+marinating time) | Cook time: 10 minutes | Servings: 4

Thai Coconut Curry Shrimp

Ingredients:
- 1 pound large shrimp, peeled and deveined

- 1 can (13.5 oz) coconut milk

- 2 tablespoons red curry paste

- 1 tablespoon fish sauce

- 1 tablespoon coconut sugar

- 1 red bell pepper, sliced

- 1 zucchini, sliced

- Fresh cilantro for garnish

- Cooked brown rice for serving

Instructions:
1. Heat coconut milk over medium heat in a wok or large skillet.

2. Stir in red curry paste, fish sauce, and coconut sugar.

3. Add shrimp, red bell pepper, and zucchini to the wok and simmer for 5-7 minutes until the shrimp are cooked.

4. Garnish Thai Coconut Curry Shrimp with fresh cilantro and serve over cooked brown rice.

Nutrition:
Calories - 280 | Protein - 20g | Carbs - 15g | Fat - 16g | Fiber - 3g

Prep time: 10 minutes | Cook time: 10 minutes | Servings: 4

Blackened Snapper with Mango Salsa

Ingredients:
- 4 snapper fillets

- 2 tablespoons blackened seasoning

- 2 tablespoons olive oil

- Mango Salsa:

  - 1 ripe mango, diced

  - 1/2 red onion, finely chopped

  - 1/4 cup fresh cilantro, chopped

  - Juice of 1 lime

  - Salt and black pepper to taste

Instructions:
1. Preheat the grill or a grill pan to medium-high heat.

2. Rub snapper fillets with blackened seasoning and drizzle with olive oil.

3. Grill the snapper for 3-4 minutes per side or until it's cooked through.

4. Mix diced mango, chopped red onion, cilantro, lime juice, salt, and black pepper to make the salsa in a bowl.

5. Top the Blackened Snapper with Mango Salsa before serving.

Nutrition:
Calories - 250 | Protein - 25g | Carbs - 15g | Fat - 10g | Fiber - 2g

Prep time: 15 minutes | Cook time: 8 minutes | Servings: 4

Pesto Grilled Shrimp Skewers

Ingredients:
- 1 pound large shrimp, peeled and deveined

- 1/4 cup pesto sauce

- 1 tablespoon olive oil

- 1 lemon, sliced

- Wooden skewers soaked in water

- Fresh basil for garnish

Instructions:
1. Preheat the grill to medium-high heat.

2. In a bowl, toss shrimp with pesto sauce and olive oil until evenly coated.

3. Thread shrimp onto soaked skewers, alternating with lemon slices.

4. Grill the shrimp skewers for 2-3 minutes per side or until they are cooked through.

5. Garnish Pesto Grilled Shrimp Skewers with fresh basil before serving.

Nutrition:
Calories - 180 | Protein - 20g | Carbs - 5g | Fat - 10g | Fiber - 1g

Prep time: 10 minutes | Cook time: 6 minutes | Servings: 4

Baked Lemon Dill Cod

Ingredients:
- 4 cod fillets

- 2 tablespoons olive oil

- 1 tablespoon lemon juice

- 1 teaspoon dried dill

- 1 teaspoon garlic powder

- Lemon slices for garnish

- Fresh dill for garnish

- Salt and black pepper to taste

Instructions:
1. Preheat the oven to 400°F (200°C).

2. Place cod fillets on a baking sheet lined with parchment paper.

3. Whisk together olive oil, lemon juice, dried dill, garlic powder, salt, and black pepper in a bowl.

4. Brush each cod fillet with the lemon dill mixture.

5. Bake in the preheated oven for 12-15 minutes or until the cod is flaky and cooked through.

6. Garnish Baked Lemon Dill Cod with lemon slices and fresh dill before serving.

Nutrition:
Calories - 220 | Protein - 25g | Carbs - 1g | Fat - 12g | Fiber - 0.5g

Prep time: 10 minutes | Cook time: 15 minutes | Servings: 4

Spicy Sriracha Glazed Salmon

Ingredients:
- 4 salmon fillets

- 2 tablespoons Sriracha sauce

- 1 tablespoon honey

- 1 tablespoon soy sauce

- 1 teaspoon sesame oil

- 1 teaspoon minced garlic

- Sesame seeds for garnish

- Green onions for garnish

Instructions:
1. Preheat the oven to 400°F (200°C).

2. Whisk together Sriracha sauce, honey, soy sauce, sesame oil, and minced garlic in a bowl.

3. Place salmon fillets on a baking sheet lined with parchment paper.

4. Brush each salmon fillet with the Sriracha glaze.

5. Bake in the preheated oven for 12-15 minutes or until the salmon is cooked through.

6. Before serving, Garnish Spicy Sriracha Glazed Salmon with sesame seeds and sliced green onions.

Nutrition:
Calories - 280 | Protein - 25g | Carbs - 10g | Fat - 15g | Fiber - 1g

Prep time: 10 minutes | Cook time: 15 minutes | Servings: 4

Chapter 4. SOUPS.

Hearty Lentil and Vegetable Soup

Ingredients:
- 1 cup dry green lentils, rinsed

- 1 onion, diced

- 2 carrots, chopped

- 2 celery stalks, chopped

- 3 cloves garlic, minced

- 1 can (14 oz) diced tomatoes

- 6 cups vegetable broth

- 1 teaspoon ground cumin

- 1 teaspoon smoked paprika

- 1 bay leaf

- Salt and black pepper to taste

- Fresh parsley for garnish

Instructions:
1. Combine lentils, onion, carrots, celery, garlic, diced tomatoes, vegetable broth, cumin, smoked paprika, and bay leaf in a large pot.

2. Bring the soup to a boil, then reduce heat and simmer for 25-30 minutes or until lentils and vegetables are tender.

3. Season with salt and black pepper to taste.

4. Remove the bay leaf before serving.

5. Garnish Hearty Lentil and Vegetable Soup with fresh parsley.

Nutrition:
Calories - 220 | Protein - 15g | Carbs - 40g | Fat - 1g | Fiber - 15g

Prep time: 10 minutes | Cook time: 30 minutes | Servings: 6

Tomato Basil Quinoa Soup

Ingredients:
- 1 cup quinoa, rinsed

- 1 onion, finely chopped

- 2 carrots, diced

- 2 celery stalks, sliced

- 3 cloves garlic, minced

- 1 can (28 oz) crushed tomatoes

- 6 cups vegetable broth

- 1 teaspoon dried basil

- 1/2 teaspoon dried oregano

- Salt and black pepper to taste

- Fresh basil leaves for garnish

Instructions:
1. Combine a large pot of quinoa, onion, carrots, celery, garlic, crushed tomatoes, vegetable broth, dried basil, and dried oregano.

2. Bring the soup to a boil, then reduce heat and simmer for 15-20 minutes or until quinoa and vegetables are cooked.

3. Season with salt and black pepper to taste.

4. Garnish Tomato Basil Quinoa Soup with fresh basil leaves before serving.

Nutrition:
Calories - 250 | Protein - 8g | Carbs - 50g | Fat - 2g | Fiber - 8g

Prep time: 10 minutes | Cook time: 20 minutes | Servings: 6

Spicy Black Bean and Kale Soup

Ingredients:
- 2 cans (15 oz each) black beans, drained and rinsed

- 1 onion, diced

- 2 carrots, grated

- 3 cloves garlic, minced

- 4 cups kale, chopped

- 1 can (14 oz) diced tomatoes with green chilies

- 6 cups vegetable broth

- 1 teaspoon ground cumin

- 1/2 teaspoon chili powder

- Salt and black pepper to taste

- Avocado slices for garnish

Instructions:

1. Combine black beans, onion, carrots, garlic, kale, diced tomatoes with green chilies, vegetable broth, ground cumin, and chili powder in a large pot.

2. Bring the soup to a boil, then reduce heat and simmer for 15-20 minutes or until vegetables are tender.

3. Season with salt and black pepper to taste.

4. Serve Spicy Black Bean and Kale Soup with avocado slices on top.

Nutrition:

Calories - 230 | Protein - 12g | Carbs - 40g | Fat - 2g | Fiber - 12g

Prep time: 15 minutes | Cook time: 20 minutes | Servings: 6

Lemon Garlic Chicken and Rice Soup

Ingredients:

- 1 lb boneless, skinless chicken breasts, shredded

- 1 cup white rice, uncooked

- 1 onion, finely chopped

- 3 carrots, sliced

- 3 celery stalks, diced

- 4 cloves garlic, minced

- 8 cups chicken broth

- 1 teaspoon dried thyme

- 1/2 teaspoon turmeric

- Juice of 2 lemons

- Salt and black pepper to taste

- Fresh parsley for garnish

Instructions:
1. In a large pot, combine shredded chicken, white rice, onion, carrots, celery, garlic, chicken broth, dried thyme, and turmeric.

2. Bring the soup to a boil, then reduce heat and simmer for 20-25 minutes or until rice is cooked and vegetables are tender.

3. Stir in the lemon juice and season with salt and black pepper to taste.

4. Garnish Lemon Garlic Chicken and Rice Soup with fresh parsley before serving.

Nutrition:
Calories - 300 | Protein - 25g | Carbs - 40g | Fat - 3g | Fiber - 3g

Prep time: 15 minutes | Cook time: 25 minutes | Servings: 6

Chickpea and Spinach Soup

Ingredients:
- 2 cans (15 oz each) chickpeas, drained and rinsed

- 1 onion, diced

- 2 carrots, chopped

- 3 cloves garlic, minced

- 4 cups baby spinach

- 1 can (14 oz) diced tomatoes

- 6 cups vegetable broth

- 1 teaspoon dried oregano

- 1/2 teaspoon ground cumin

- Juice of 1 lemon

- Salt and black pepper to taste

- Feta cheese for garnish (optional)

Instructions:

1. Combine chickpeas, onion, carrots, garlic, baby spinach, diced tomatoes, vegetable broth, dried oregano, and ground cumin in a large pot.

2. Bring the soup to a boil, then reduce heat and simmer for 15-20 minutes or until vegetables are tender.

3. Stir in the lemon juice and season with salt and black pepper to taste.

4. Serve Mediterranean Chickpea and Spinach Soup hot, garnished with crumbled feta cheese if desired.

Nutrition:

Calories - 250 | Protein - 12g | Carbs - 40g | Fat - 5g | Fiber - 10g

Prep time: 15 minutes | Cook time: 20 minutes | Servings: 6

Thai Coconut Curry Lentil Soup

Ingredients:

- 1 cup dry red lentils, rinsed

- 1 onion, finely chopped

- 2 carrots, sliced

- 3 cloves garlic, minced

- 2 tablespoons red curry paste

- 1 can (14 oz) coconut milk

- 6 cups vegetable broth

- 1 tablespoon soy sauce

- Juice of 1 lime

- Fresh cilantro for garnish

- Red chili flakes for spice (optional)

Instructions:

1. In a large pot, Combine red lentils, onion, carrots, garlic, red curry paste, coconut milk, vegetable broth, and soy sauce.

2. Bring the soup to a boil, then reduce heat and simmer for 15-20 minutes or until lentils are cooked.

3. Stir in the lime juice and add red chili flakes for extra spice if desired.

4. Garnish Thai Coconut Curry Lentil Soup with fresh cilantro before serving.

Nutrition:
Calories - 280 | Protein - 15g | Carbs - 30g | Fat - 12g | Fiber - 8g

Prep time: 10 minutes | Cook time: 20 minutes | Servings: 6

Creamy Sweet Potato and Red Pepper Soup

Ingredients:
- 2 large sweet potatoes, peeled and diced

- 2 red bell peppers, chopped

- 1 onion, diced

- 3 cloves garlic, minced

- 4 cups vegetable broth

- 1 can (14 oz) coconut milk

- 1 teaspoon ground cumin

- 1/2 teaspoon smoked paprika

- Salt and black pepper to taste

- Fresh chives for garnish

Instructions:
1. Combine sweet potatoes, red bell peppers, onion, garlic, vegetable broth, coconut milk, ground cumin, and smoked paprika in a large pot.

2. Bring the soup to a boil, then reduce heat and simmer for 20-25 minutes or until sweet potatoes are tender.

3. Use an immersion blender to puree the soup until smooth.

4. Season with salt and black pepper to taste.

5. Garnish Creamy Sweet Potato and Red Pepper Soup with fresh chives before serving.

Nutrition:
Calories - 280 | Protein - 5g | Carbs - 35g | Fat - 15g | Fiber - 6g

Prep time: 15 minutes | Cook time: 25 minutes | Servings: 6

Roasted Red Pepper and Lentil Soup

Ingredients:
- 1 cup dry red lentils, rinsed

- 3 red bell peppers, roasted and chopped

- 1 onion, finely chopped

- 3 cloves garlic, minced

- 6 cups vegetable broth

- 1 teaspoon ground cumin

- 1/2 teaspoon smoked paprika

- Juice of 1 lemon

- Salt and black pepper to taste

- Fresh parsley for garnish

Instructions:
1. Combine red lentils, roasted red peppers, onion, garlic, vegetable broth, ground cumin, and smoked paprika in a large pot.

2. Bring the soup to a boil, then reduce heat and simmer for 15-20 minutes or until lentils are cooked.

3. Stir in the lemon juice and season with salt and black pepper to taste.

4. Garnish Roasted Red Pepper and Lentil Soup with fresh parsley before serving.

Nutrition:
Calories - 250 | Protein - 12g | Carbs - 40g | Fat - 3g | Fiber - 10g

Prep time: 10 minutes | Cook time: 20 minutes | Servings: 6

Chicken, Barley, and Mushroom Soup

Ingredients:
- 1 lb chicken breasts, cooked and shredded

- 1 cup pearl barley, cooked

- 1 onion, diced

- 2 carrots, sliced

- 2 celery stalks, diced

- 3 cups mushrooms, sliced

- 3 cloves garlic, minced

- 8 cups chicken broth

- 1 teaspoon dried thyme

- 1/2 teaspoon rosemary

- Salt and black pepper to taste

- Fresh dill for garnish

Instructions:
1. Combine shredded chicken, cooked barley, onion, carrots, celery, mushrooms, garlic, chicken broth, dried thyme, and rosemary in a large pot.

2. Bring the soup to a boil, then reduce heat and simmer for 20-25 minutes or until vegetables are tender.

3. Season with salt and black pepper to taste.

4. Garnish Chicken, Barley, and Mushroom Soup with fresh dill before serving.

Nutrition:
Calories - 300 | Protein - 25g | Carbs - 35g | Fat - 5g | Fiber - 8g

Prep time: 20 minutes | Cook time: 25 minutes | Servings: 6

Cabbage and Sausage Detox Soup

Ingredients:
- 1 lb smoked beef sausage, sliced

- 1 head cabbage, shredded

- 2 onions, diced

- 3 carrots, julienned

- 3 cloves garlic, minced

- 1 can (14 oz) diced tomatoes

- 8 cups beef broth

- 1 teaspoon turmeric

- 1/2 teaspoon cayenne pepper

- Salt and black pepper to taste

- Fresh parsley for garnish

Instructions:

1. In a large pot, sauté sliced sausage until browned.

2. Add shredded cabbage, diced onions, julienned carrots, minced garlic, diced tomatoes, beef broth, turmeric, and cayenne pepper.

3. Bring the soup to a boil, then reduce heat and simmer for 20-25 minutes or until vegetables are cooked.

4. Season with salt and black pepper to taste.

5. Garnish Cabbage and Sausage Detox Soup with fresh parsley before serving.

Nutrition:

Calories - 280 | Protein - 15g | Carbs - 20g | Fat - 18g | Fiber - 6g

Prep time: 15 minutes | Cook time: 25 minutes | Servings: 6

Scandinavian Salmon Soup

Ingredients:

- 1 lb salmon fillet, skin-on, cut into chunks

- 1 leek, sliced

- 2 carrots, diced

- 2 potatoes, peeled and cubed

- 1 celery stalk, sliced

- 1 onion, finely chopped

- 3 cups fish or vegetable broth

- 1 cup milk

- 1/2 cup heavy cream

- 2 tablespoons butter

- 1 bay leaf

- 1 teaspoon dill, dried

- Salt and white pepper to taste

- Fresh parsley for garnish

Instructions:

1. In a large pot, melt butter and sauté leek, carrots, celery, and onion until softened.

2. Add fish or vegetable broth, milk, heavy cream, bay leaf, and dried dill. Bring to a simmer.

3. Gently add salmon chunks to the pot, ensuring the skin is facing down.

4. Simmer for 10-15 minutes or until salmon is cooked through.

5. Season with salt and white pepper to taste.

6. Garnish Scandinavian Salmon Soup with fresh parsley before serving.

Nutrition:

Calories - 300 | Protein - 25g | Carbs - 20g | Fat - 15g | Fiber - 3g

Prep time: 15 minutes | Cook time: 20 minutes | Servings: 4

Roasted Butternut Squash with Sage

Ingredients:
- 1 medium butternut squash, peeled and diced

- 2 tablespoons olive oil

- 1 tablespoon fresh sage, chopped

- 1 teaspoon maple syrup

- Salt and black pepper to taste

Instructions:
1. Preheat the oven to 400°F (200°C).

2. Toss butternut squash with olive oil, chopped sage, maple syrup, salt, and black pepper in a bowl.

3. Spread the squash evenly on a baking sheet.

4. Roast in the oven for 25-30 minutes or until the edges are golden brown and caramelized.

5. Remove from the oven and serve the Roasted Butternut Squash with Sage as a side dish.

Nutrition:
Calories - 120 | Protein - 2g | Carbs - 25g | Fat - 4g | Fiber - 4g

Prep time: 10 minutes | Cook time: 30 minutes | Servings: 4

Harissa Spiced Roasted Eggplant

Ingredients:
- 2 large eggplants, sliced

- 3 tablespoons olive oil

- 2 tablespoons harissa paste

- 1 teaspoon ground cumin

- 1 teaspoon smoked paprika

- Salt and black pepper to taste

- Fresh cilantro for garnish

Instructions:
1. Preheat the oven to 400°F (200°C).

2. Add olive oil, harissa paste, ground cumin, smoked paprika, salt, and black pepper in a bowl.

3. Brush the eggplant slices with the harissa mixture, ensuring both sides are coated.

4. Place the eggplant on a baking sheet and roast in the oven for 20-25 minutes or until tender.

5. Garnish the Harissa Spiced Roasted Eggplant with fresh cilantro before serving.

Nutrition:
Calories - 150 | Protein - 3g | Carbs - 20g | Fat - 8g | Fiber - 10g

Prep time: 15 minutes | Cook time: 25 minutes | Servings: 4

Spinach and Feta Stuffed Mushrooms

Ingredients:
- 12 large mushrooms, stems removed

- 1 cup fresh spinach, chopped

- 1/2 cup feta cheese, crumbled

- 2 tablespoons olive oil

- 2 cloves garlic, minced

- 1 teaspoon dried oregano

- Salt and black pepper to taste

Instructions:
1. Preheat the oven to 375°F (190°C).

2. In a skillet, heat olive oil and sauté garlic until fragrant.

3. Add chopped spinach and cook until wilted.

4. Mix the sautéed spinach with crumbled feta, dried oregano, salt, and black pepper in a bowl.

5. Stuff each mushroom cap with the Spinach and Feta mixture.

6. Place stuffed mushrooms on a baking sheet and bake for 15-18 minutes or until mushrooms are tender.

7. Serve the Spinach and Feta Stuffed Mushrooms as a delightful appetizer.

Nutrition:
Calories - 90 | Protein - 4g | Carbs - 6g | Fat - 6g | Fiber - 2g

Prep time: 20 minutes | Cook time: 15 minutes | Servings: 6

Garlic Lemon, Green Bean Almondine

Ingredients:
- 1 lb green beans, trimmed

- 2 tablespoons olive oil

- 3 cloves garlic, minced

- Zest of 1 lemon

- 1/2 cup sliced almonds

- Salt and black pepper to taste

- Fresh parsley for garnish

Instructions:
1. Blanch green beans in boiling water for 2-3 minutes, then transfer to an ice bath to stop cooking.

2. In a skillet, heat olive oil over medium heat. Add minced garlic and sauté until fragrant.

3. Add lemon zest and sliced almonds to the skillet, cooking until almonds are lightly toasted.

4. Toss the blanched green beans into the skillet, coating them with the garlic-lemon-almond mixture.

5. Season with salt and black pepper, garnish with fresh parsley and serve the Garlic Lemon, Green Bean, and Almondine.

Nutrition:
Calories - 120 | Protein - 4g | Carbs - 10g | Fat - 8g | Fiber - 5g

Prep time: 15 minutes | Cook time: 10 minutes | Servings: 4

Turmeric Roasted Broccoli

Ingredients:
- 1 lb broccoli florets

- 2 tablespoons olive oil

- 1 teaspoon ground turmeric

- 1/2 teaspoon smoked paprika

- Salt and black pepper to taste

- Lemon wedges for serving

Instructions:
1. Preheat the oven to 425°F (220°C).

2. Toss broccoli florets with olive oil, ground turmeric, smoked paprika, salt, and black pepper.

3. Spread the seasoned broccoli on a baking sheet.

4. Roast in the oven for 20-25 minutes or until broccoli is crispy at the edges.

5. Squeeze lemon wedges over the turmeric-roasted broccoli before serving.

Nutrition:
Calories - 90 | Protein - 5g | Carbs - 8g | Fat - 6g | Fiber - 4g

Prep time: 10 minutes | Cook time: 25 minutes | Servings: 4

Honey Dijon Glazed Roasted Beets

Ingredients:
- 4 medium beets, peeled and diced

- 2 tablespoons olive oil

- 2 tablespoons honey

- 1 tablespoon Dijon mustard

- Salt and black pepper to taste

- Fresh thyme for garnish

Instructions:
1. Preheat the oven to 400°F (200°C).

2. Toss diced beets with olive oil, honey, Dijon mustard, salt, and black pepper in a bowl.

3. Spread the coated beets on a baking sheet.

4. Roast in the oven for 30-35 minutes or until beets are tender.

5. Garnish the Honey Dijon Glazed Roasted Beets with fresh thyme before serving.

Nutrition:
Calories - 120 | Protein - 2g | Carbs - 20g | Fat - 5g | Fiber - 4g

Prep time: 15 minutes | Cook time: 35 minutes | Servings: 4

Sesame Ginger Snap Pea Stir-Fry

Ingredients:
- 1 lb snap peas, trimmed

- 2 tablespoons sesame oil

- 1 tablespoon soy sauce

- 1 teaspoon fresh ginger, grated

- 1 clove garlic, minced

- 1 tablespoon sesame seeds

- Green onions for garnish

Instructions:
1. Heat sesame oil over medium-high heat in a wok or skillet.

2. Add snap peas, grated ginger, and minced garlic, stir-frying for 3-4 minutes until peas are tender-crisp.

3. Drizzle soy sauce over the snap peas, tossing to coat evenly.

4. Sprinkle sesame seeds and garnish with chopped green onions before serving the Sesame Ginger Snap Pea Stir-Fry.

Nutrition:
Calories - 80 | Protein - 3g | Carbs - 8g | Fat - 5g | Fiber - 3g

Prep time: 10 minutes | Cook time: 5 minutes | Servings: 4

Ginger Sesame Stir-Fried Bok Choy

Ingredients:
- 4 baby bok choy, halved

- 2 tablespoons sesame oil

- 1 tablespoon soy sauce

- 1 teaspoon fresh ginger, minced

- 1 clove garlic, minced

- 1 tablespoon sesame seeds

- Red pepper flakes for spice (optional)

Instructions:
1. Heat sesame oil over medium-high heat in a wok or skillet.

2. Add bok choy halves, ginger, and garlic, stir-frying for 3-4 minutes until bok choy is tender-crisp.

3. Drizzle soy sauce over the bok choy and toss to coat evenly.

4. Sprinkle sesame seeds and red pepper flakes (if using) over the Ginger Sesame Stir-Fried Bok Choy before serving.

Nutrition:
Calories - 60 | Protein - 3g | Carbs - 5g | Fat - 4g | Fiber - 2g

Prep time: 10 minutes | Cook time: 5 minutes | Servings: 4

Mediterranean Stuffed Eggplants

Ingredients:
- 2 large eggplants, halved

- 1 cup cherry tomatoes, halved

- 1/2 cup crumbled feta cheese

- 1/4 cup Kalamata olives, sliced

- 2 tablespoons olive oil

- 1 teaspoon dried oregano

- Salt and black pepper to taste

- Fresh parsley for garnish

Instructions:
1. Preheat the oven to 375°F (190°C).

2. Scoop out the center of each eggplant half, leaving a shell.

3. Mix cherry tomatoes, feta cheese, Kalamata olives, olive oil, dried oregano, salt, and black pepper in a bowl.

4. Stuff each eggplant half with the Mediterranean mixture.

5. Place the stuffed eggplants on a baking sheet and bake for 25-30 minutes or until eggplants are tender.

6. Garnish the Mediterranean Stuffed Eggplants with fresh parsley before serving.

Nutrition:
Calories - 180 | Protein - 6g | Carbs - 15g | Fat - 12g | Fiber - 8g

Prep time: 15 minutes | Cook time: 30 minutes | Servings: 4

Spicy Kale and Chickpea Sauté

Ingredients:
- 4 cups kale, chopped

- 1 can (15 oz) chickpeas, drained and rinsed

- 2 tablespoons olive oil

- 1 clove garlic, minced

- 1 teaspoon smoked paprika

- 1/2 teaspoon cayenne pepper

- Salt and black pepper to taste

- Lemon wedges for serving

Instructions:
1. In a large skillet, heat olive oil over medium heat.

2. Add minced garlic, kale, and chickpeas, sautéing until kale is wilted and chickpeas are heated through.

3. Sprinkle smoked paprika, cayenne pepper, salt, and black pepper over the kale-chickpea mixture.

4. Squeeze lemon wedges over the Spicy Kale and Chickpea Sauté before serving.

Nutrition:
Calories - 200 | Protein - 8g | Carbs - 25g | Fat - 8g | Fiber - 8g

Prep time: 10 minutes | Cook time: 10 minutes | Servings: 4

Cumin Roasted Sweet Potato Wedges

Ingredients:
- 2 large sweet potatoes, cut into wedges

- 2 tablespoons olive oil

- 1 teaspoon ground cumin

- 1/2 teaspoon smoked paprika

- Salt and black pepper to taste

- Fresh cilantro for garnish

Instructions:
1. Preheat the oven to 400°F (200°C).

2. Toss sweet potato wedges with olive oil, ground cumin, smoked paprika, salt, and black pepper.

3. Spread the seasoned sweet potatoes on a baking sheet.

4. Roast in the oven for 25-30 minutes or until sweet potatoes are tender.

5. Garnish the Cumin Roasted Sweet Potato Wedges with fresh cilantro before serving.

Nutrition:
Calories - 150 | Protein - 2g | Carbs - 25g | Fat - 6g | Fiber - 4g

Prep time: 15 minutes | Cook time: 30 minutes | Servings:* 4

Greek-Style Stuffed Tomatoes

Ingredients:
- 4 large tomatoes, tops removed and insides scooped out

- 1 cup quinoa, cooked

- 1/2 cup crumbled feta cheese

- 1/4 cup red onion, finely chopped

- 2 tablespoons Kalamata olives, sliced

- 2 tablespoons fresh dill, chopped

- 2 tablespoons olive oil

- Salt and black pepper to taste

Instructions:
1. Preheat the oven to 375°F (190°C).

2. Mix cooked quinoa, feta cheese, red onion, Kalamata olives, fresh dill, olive oil, salt, and black pepper in a bowl.

3. Stuff each tomato with the Greek-style quinoa mixture.

4. Place the stuffed tomatoes in a baking dish and bake for 15-20 minutes or until the tomatoes are tender.

5. Garnish the Greek-style stuffed Tomatoes with an extra sprinkle of fresh dill before serving.

Nutrition:
Calories - 180 | Protein - 6g | Carbs - 25g | Fat - 8g | Fiber - 4g

Prep time: 15 minutes | Cook time: 15-20 minutes | Servings: 4

Berry Blast Yogurt Parfait

Ingredients:
- 1 cup Greek yogurt

- 1/2 cup mixed berries (blueberries, strawberries, raspberries)

- 2 tablespoons granola

- 1 tablespoon honey

- Fresh mint leaves for garnish

Instructions:
1. In a glass or bowl, layer Greek yogurt.

2. Add a layer of mixed berries on top.

3. Sprinkle granola over the berries.

4. Drizzle honey over the parfait.

5. Repeat the layers until the glass is filled.

6. Garnish with fresh mint leaves.

7. Enjoy your Berry Blast Yogurt Parfait!

Nutrition:
Calories - 250 | Protein - 15g | Carbs - 30g | Fat - 10g | Fiber - 5g

Prep time: 10 minutes | Servings: 1

Dark Chocolate-Dipped Strawberries

Ingredients:
- 1 cup fresh strawberries, washed and dried

- 1/2 cup dark chocolate chips

- 1 teaspoon coconut oil

- Chopped nuts or shredded coconut (optional)

Instructions:
1. In a microwave-safe bowl, melt dark chocolate chips with coconut oil in 30-second intervals, stirring until smooth.

2. Dip each strawberry into the melted chocolate, coating about two-thirds of the berry.

3. Place dipped strawberries on a parchment-lined tray.

4. Optional: Sprinkle chopped nuts or shredded coconut over the chocolate.

5. Refrigerate until the chocolate hardens.

6. Enjoy your Dark Chocolate-Dipped Strawberries!

Nutrition:
Calories - 120 | Protein - 2g | Carbs - 15g | Fat - 7g | Fiber - 3g

Prep time: 15 minutes | Servings:* 4

Cinnamon Apple Slices with Almond Butter

Ingredients:
- 2 medium apples, sliced

- 2 tablespoons almond butter

- 1 teaspoon ground cinnamon

- Sliced almonds for garnish

Instructions:
1. Arrange apple slices on a plate.

2. Warm almond butter slightly and drizzle over the apple slices.

3. Sprinkle ground cinnamon over the apples.

4. Garnish with sliced almonds.

5. Enjoy your Cinnamon Apple Slices with Almond Butter!

Nutrition:
Calories - 200 | Protein - 4g | Carbs - 25g | Fat - 10g | Fiber - 6g

Prep time: 5 minutes | Servings: 2

Greek Yogurt and Honey Frozen Blueberry Bites

Ingredients:
- 1 cup Greek yogurt

- 1 cup fresh blueberries

- 2 tablespoons honey

Instructions:
1. In a bowl, mix Greek yogurt and honey until well combined.

2. Dip each blueberry into the yogurt mixture, coating it entirely.

3. Place the coated blueberries on a parchment-lined tray.

4. Freeze until solid.

5. Enjoy your Greek Yogurt and Honey Frozen Blueberry Bites!

Nutrition:
Calories - 150 | Protein - 10g | Carbs - 20g | Fat - 5g | Fiber - 3g

Prep time: 10 minutes | Freeze time: 2 hours | Servings: 4

Avocado Chocolate Mousse

Ingredients:
- 2 ripe avocados

- 1/4 cup unsweetened cocoa powder

- 1/4 cup maple syrup

- 1 teaspoon vanilla extract

- A pinch of salt

- Fresh berries for garnish

Instructions:
1. Combine avocados, cocoa powder, maple syrup, vanilla extract, and a pinch of salt in a blender.

2. Blend until smooth and creamy.

3. Spoon the mousse into serving glasses.

4. Refrigerate for at least 30 minutes.

5. Garnish with fresh berries before serving.

6. Enjoy your Avocado Chocolate Mousse!

Nutrition:
Calories - 180 | Protein - 3g | Carbs - 20g | Fat - 12g | Fiber - 7g

Prep time: 10 minutes | Chill time: 30 minutes | Servings: 2

Roasted Chickpeas with Smoky Paprika

Ingredients:
- 1 can (15 oz) chickpeas, drained and rinsed

- 1 tablespoon olive oil

- 1 teaspoon smoked paprika

- 1/2 teaspoon garlic powder

- 1/2 teaspoon cumin

- Salt and pepper to taste

Instructions:
1. Preheat the oven to 400°F (200°C).

2. Pat dry the chickpeas with a paper towel to remove excess moisture.

3. Toss chickpeas with olive oil, smoked paprika, garlic powder, cumin, salt, and pepper in a bowl.

4. Spread the chickpeas on a baking sheet in a single layer.

5. Roast for 20-25 minutes or until crispy, shaking the pan halfway through.

6. Let cool before serving.

7. Enjoy your Roasted Chickpeas with Smoky Paprika!

Nutrition:
Calories - 150 | Protein - 6g | Carbs - 20g | Fat - 5g | Fiber - 6g

Prep time: 5 minutes | Cook time: 25 minutes | Servings: 4

Almond and Chia Seed Energy Bites

Ingredients:
- 1 cup rolled oats

- 1/2 cup almond butter

- 1/4 cup honey

- 1/4 cup chia seeds

- 1/2 teaspoon vanilla extract

- A pinch of salt

- Shredded coconut for rolling (optional)

Instructions:
1. Mix rolled oats, almond butter, honey, chia seeds, vanilla extract, and a pinch of salt in a bowl.

2. Refrigerate the mixture for 15-20 minutes to firm up.

3. Roll the mixture into bite-sized balls.

4. Optional: Roll the balls in shredded coconut.

5. Refrigerate for an additional 30 minutes.

6. Enjoy your Almond and Chia Seed Energy Bites!

Nutrition:
Calories - 120 | Protein - 4g | Carbs - 15g | Fat - 6g | Fiber - 3g

Prep time: 15 minutes | Chill time: 30 minutes | Servings: 12

Baked Sweet Potato Chips with Rosemary

Ingredients:
- 2 medium sweet potatoes, thinly sliced

- 2 tablespoons olive oil

- 1 teaspoon dried rosemary

- Salt to taste

Instructions:
1. Preheat the oven to 400°F (200°C).

2. Toss sweet potato slices with olive oil, dried rosemary, and salt in a bowl.

3. Arrange the slices on a baking sheet in a single layer.

4. Bake for 15-20 minutes or until crispy, flipping halfway through.

5. Let cool before serving.

6. Enjoy your Baked Sweet Potato Chips with Rosemary!

Nutrition:
Calories - 120 | Protein - 1g | Carbs - 20g | Fat - 4g | Fiber - 3g

Prep time: 10 minutes | Bake time: 20 minutes | Servings: 4

Mango Salsa with Whole Grain Pita Chips

Ingredients:
- 2 ripe mangoes, diced

- 1/2 red onion, finely chopped

- 1 jalapeño, seeded and minced

- 1/4 cup fresh cilantro, chopped

- Juice of 1 lime

- Salt to taste

- Whole grain pita chips for serving

Instructions:
1. Combine diced mangoes, chopped red onion, minced jalapeño, and chopped cilantro in a bowl.

2. Squeeze lime juice over the mixture and add salt to taste.

3. Mix well and refrigerate for at least 30 minutes.

4. Serve the Mango Salsa with whole-grain pita chips.

5. Enjoy your Mango Salsa with Whole Grain Pita Chips!

Nutrition:
Calories - 100 | Protein - 2g | Carbs - 25g | Fat - 1g | Fiber - 4g

Prep time: 15 minutes | Chill time: 30 minutes | Servings: 4

Vanilla Chia Pudding with Fresh Berries

Ingredients:
- 1/4 cup chia seeds

- 1 cup unsweetened almond milk

- 1 tablespoon pure vanilla extract

- 1 tablespoon maple syrup

- Fresh berries for topping

Instructions:
1. Mix chia seeds, almond milk, vanilla extract, and maple syrup in a jar.

2. Stir well and refrigerate overnight or for at least 4 hours.

3. Before serving, stir the pudding to ensure a smooth consistency.

4. Top with fresh berries before serving.

5. Enjoy your Vanilla Chia Pudding with Fresh Berries!

Nutrition:
Calories - 150 | Protein - 4g | Carbs - 20g | Fat - 6g | Fiber - 8g

Prep time: 5 minutes | Chill time: 4 hours | Servings: 2

Pistachio and Cranberry Trail Mix

Ingredients:
- 1/2 cup pistachios

- 1/2 cup dried cranberries

- 1/4 cup almonds

- 1/4 cup walnuts

- 1/4 cup dark chocolate chips (optional)

Instructions:
1. In a bowl, combine pistachios, dried cranberries, almonds, walnuts, and dark chocolate chips if using.

2. Toss until well mixed.

3. Portion into snack-sized containers.

4. Enjoy your Pistachio and Cranberry Trail Mix!

Nutrition:
Calories - 200 | Protein - 5g | Carbs - 20g | Fat - 12g | Fiber - 4g

Prep time: 5 minutes | Servings: 4

Baked Cinnamon Banana Chips

Ingredients:
- 2 ripe bananas

- 1 tablespoon coconut oil, melted

- 1 teaspoon ground cinnamon

Instructions:
1. Preheat the oven to 200°F (95°C).

2. Thinly slice the bananas.

3. Toss banana slices with melted coconut oil and ground cinnamon in a bowl.

4. Arrange the slices on a parchment-lined baking sheet.

5. Bake for 2-3 hours or until the chips are crispy.

6. Let cool before serving.

7. Enjoy your Baked Cinnamon Banana Chips!

Nutrition:
Calories - 80 | Protein - 1g | Carbs - 20g | Fat - 3g | Fiber - 3g

Prep time: 10 minutes | Bake time: 2-3 hours | Servings: 2

Caprese Skewers with Balsamic Glaze

Ingredients:
- Cherry tomatoes

- Fresh mozzarella balls

- Fresh basil leaves

- Balsamic glaze

Instructions:
1. Thread cherry tomatoes, fresh mozzarella balls, and fresh basil leaves onto skewers.

2. Arrange the skewers on a serving platter.

3. Drizzle balsamic glaze over the skewers.

4. Serve the Caprese Skewers with Balsamic Glaze.

5. Enjoy this delightful appetizer!

Nutrition:
Calories - 90 | Protein - 5g | Carbs - 3g | Fat - 6g | Fiber - 1g

Prep time: 10 minutes | Servings: 2

Coconut and Berry Smoothie Bowl

Ingredients:
- 1 cup mixed berries (strawberries, blueberries, raspberries)

- 1/2 banana

- 1/2 cup coconut milk

- 1/4 cup rolled oats

- 1 tablespoon shredded coconut

- Chia seeds and sliced almonds for topping

Instructions:
1. In a blender, blend mixed berries, banana, coconut milk, and rolled oats until smooth.

2. Pour the smoothie into a bowl.

3. Top with shredded coconut, chia seeds, and sliced almonds.

4. Enjoy your Coconut and Berry Smoothie Bowl!

Nutrition:
Calories - 300 | Protein - 5g | Carbs - 40g | Fat - 15g | Fiber - 8g

Prep time: 5 minutes | Servings: 2

Roasted Red Pepper Hummus with Veggie Sticks

Ingredients:
- 1 can (15 oz) chickpeas, drained and rinsed

- 1/2 cup roasted red peppers

- 1/4 cup tahini

- 2 tablespoons olive oil

- 1 clove garlic

- Juice of 1 lemon

- Carrot and cucumber sticks for dipping

Instructions:
1. Blend chickpeas, roasted red peppers, tahini, olive oil, garlic, and lemon juice until smooth in a food processor.

2. Transfer the hummus to a serving bowl.

3. Serve with carrot and cucumber sticks.

4. Enjoy your Roasted Red Pepper Hummus with Veggie Sticks!

Nutrition:
Calories - 150 | Protein - 5g | Carbs - 15g | Fat - 9g | Fiber - 5g

Prep time: 10 minutes | Servings: 4

Walnut and Date Protein Bars

Ingredients:
- 1 cup walnuts

- 1 cup pitted dates

- 1/2 cup protein powder (vanilla or chocolate flavor)

- 1/4 cup unsweetened cocoa powder

- 1 tablespoon almond butter

- A pinch of salt

Instructions:
1. In a food processor, combine walnuts, pitted dates, protein powder, cocoa powder, almond butter, and a pinch of salt.

2. Blend until the mixture forms a sticky dough.

3. Press the dough into a lined pan and refrigerate for at least 2 hours.

4. Cut into bars before serving.

5. Enjoy your Walnut and Date Protein Bars!

Nutrition:
Calories - 200 | Protein - 8g | Carbs - 20g | Fat - 12g | Fiber - 4g

Prep time: 15 minutes | Chill time: 2 hours | Servings: 8

Orange and Ginger Infused Watermelon Cubes

Ingredients:
- Watermelon, cut into cubes

- Oranges, thinly sliced

- Fresh ginger, sliced

- Mint leaves for garnish

Instructions:
1. Combine watermelon cubes, orange slices, and sliced fresh ginger in a bowl.

2. Toss gently to mix the flavors.

3. Let it sit in the refrigerator for at least 1 hour.

4. Skewer the infused watermelon cubes on toothpicks and garnish with mint leaves.

5. Serve the Orange and Ginger Infused Watermelon Cubes as a refreshing snack.

6. Enjoy the hydrating and flavorful treat!

Nutrition:
Calories - 50 | Protein - 1g | Carbs - 12g | Fat - 0g | Fiber - 1g

Greek Yogurt and Mixed Berry Popsicles

Ingredients:
- 1 cup Greek yogurt

- Mixed berries (blueberries, raspberries, strawberries)

- Honey to taste

Instructions:
1. In a bowl, mix Greek yogurt with honey to taste.

2. Spoon a layer of the yogurt mixture into popsicle molds.

3. Add a layer of mixed berries.

4. Repeat the layers until the molds are filled.

5. Insert popsicle sticks and freeze for at least 4 hours.

6. Unmold the Greek Yogurt and Mixed Berry Popsicles before serving.

7. Enjoy the cool and creamy popsicles!

Nutrition:
Calories - 80 | Protein - 5g | Carbs - 12g | Fat - 2g | Fiber - 2g

Spiced Pumpkin Seed Clusters

Ingredients:
- 1 cup pumpkin seeds

- 1 tablespoon maple syrup

- 1/2 teaspoon ground cinnamon

- 1/4 teaspoon ground nutmeg

- A pinch of sea salt

Instructions:
1. Preheat the oven to 300°F (150°C) and line a baking sheet with parchment paper.

2. Toss pumpkin seeds with maple syrup, ground cinnamon, ground nutmeg, and a pinch of sea salt in a bowl.

3. Spread the pumpkin seeds on the prepared baking sheet.

4. Bake for 20-25 minutes or until golden brown, stirring halfway through.

5. Let the Spiced Pumpkin Seed Clusters cool before serving.

6. Enjoy the crunchy and flavorful clusters!

Nutrition:
Calories - 120 | Protein - 5g | Carbs - 8g | Fat - 8g | Fiber - 2g

Dark Chocolate Avocado Truffles

Ingredients:
- 1 ripe avocado, mashed

- 1/4 cup dark cocoa powder

- 2 tablespoons maple syrup

- 1/2 teaspoon vanilla extract

- Dark chocolate chips for coating

Instructions:
1. Combine mashed avocado, dark cocoa powder, maple syrup, and vanilla extract in a bowl.

2. Mix until smooth and well combined.

3. Shape the mixture into small truffles and place them on a parchment-lined tray.

4. Freeze for 30 minutes.

5. Melt dark chocolate chips and dip each truffle to coat.

6. Place back on the tray and refrigerate until the chocolate sets.

7. Enjoy the indulgent Dark Chocolate Avocado Truffles!

Nutrition:
Calories - 60 | Protein - 1g | Carbs - 8g | Fat - 4g | Fiber - 3g

Prep time: 20 minutes | Freeze time: 30 minutes | Servings: 12

COOKING CONVERSION CHART

Oven Temperatures

FAHRENHEIT (F)	CELSIUS (C) (APPROXIMATE)
250	120
300	150
325	165
350	180
375	190
400	200
425	220
450	230

Weight Equivalents

US STANDARD	METRIC (APPROXIMATE)
½ ounce	15 g
1 ounce	30 g
2 ounces	60 g
4 ounces	115 g
8 ounces	225 g
12 ounces	340 g
16 ounces or 1 pound	455 g

Volume Equivalents (Liquid)

US STANDARD	US STANDARD (OUNCES)	METRIC (APPROXIMATE)
2 tablespoons	1 fl. oz.	30 mL
¼ cup	2 fl. oz.	60 mL
½ cup	4 fl. oz.	120 mL
1 cup	8 fl. oz.	240 mL
1½ cups	12 fl. oz.	355 mL
2 cups or 1 pint	16 fl. oz.	475 mL
4 cups or 1 quart	32 fl. oz.	1 L
1 gallon	128 fl. oz.	4 L

Volume Equivalents (Dry)

US STANDARD	METRIC (APPROXIMATE)
⅛ teaspoon	0.5 mL
¼ teaspoon	1 mL
½ teaspoon	2 mL
¾ teaspoon	4 mL
1 teaspoon	5 mL
1 tablespoon	15 mL
¼ cup	59 mL
⅓ cup	79 mL
½ cup	118 mL
⅔ cup	156 mL
¾ cup	177 mL
1 cup	235 mL
2 cups or 1 pint	475 mL
3 cups	700 mL
4 cups or 1 quart	1 L
½ gallon	2 L
1 gallon	4 L

30-DAY MEAL PLAN

Day	Breakfast	Lunch	Dinner	Snack/Dessert
1	Quinoa and Vegetable Power Bowl	Grilled Chicken and Quinoa Salad	Dijon and Honey Glazed Tilapia	Berry Blast Yogurt Parfait
2	Berry and Greek Yogurt Parfait	Spinach and Feta Turkey Burger	Citrus-Infused Mahi Mahi	Dark Chocolate-Dipped Strawberries
3	Spinach and Feta Egg Muffins	Mediterranean Stuffed Bell Peppers with Ground Beef	Cajun Spiced Catfish Fillets	Cinnamon Apple Slices with Almond Butter
4	Avocado Toast Extravaganza	Garlic and Herb Marinated Pork Tenderloin	Sesame Soy Glazed Tuna Steaks	Greek Yogurt and Honey Frozen Blueberry Bites
5	Zesty Tomato and Basil Frittata	Herb-Crusted Lamb Chops with Mint Yogurt Sauce	Coconut Lime Grilled Shrimp	Avocado Chocolate Mousse
6	Cinnamon Apple Oatmeal Elegance	Spicy Grilled Chicken Fajitas	Teriyaki Salmon Bowls	Roasted Chickpeas with Smoky Paprika

Day	Breakfast	Lunch	Dinner	Snack/Dessert
7	Smoked Salmon and Cream Cheese Bagel	Ginger Soy Glazed Beef Stir-Fry	Herb Marinated Grilled Sea Bass	Almond and Chia Seed Energy Bites
8	Sweet Potato Hash Sunrise	Cranberry Balsamic Glazed Chicken Drumsticks	Lemon Garlic Butter Scallops	Baked Sweet Potato Chips with Rosemary
9	Tropical Fruit Smoothie Bowl	Dijon Mustard and Honey Glazed Pork Chops	Chili Lime Grilled Halibut	Mango Salsa with Whole Grain Pita Chips
10	Whole Wheat Pancake Perfection	Herbed Grilled Lamb Skewers	Garlic Parmesan Crusted Tilapia	Vanilla Chia Pudding with Fresh Berries
11	Mediterranean Veggie Scramble	Chipotle Lime Grilled Chicken Wings	Almond-Crusted Baked Catfish	Pistachio and Cranberry Trail Mix
12	Blueberry Almond Breakfast Quinoa	Garlic Rosemary Roasted Leg of Lamb	Teriyaki Glazed Pineapple Salmon	Baked Cinnamon Banana Chips
13	Green Goddess	Barbecue Chicken and Quinoa Stuffed Bell	Italian Herb Marinated	Caprese Skewers with

Day	Breakfast	Lunch	Dinner	Snack/Dessert
	Breakfast Wrap	Peppers	Grilled Pork Chops	Balsamic Glaze
14	Almond Butter Banana Toast	Apple Cider Vinegar Marinated Grilled Pork Tenderloin	Apple Cider Vinegar Marinated Grilled Pork Tenderloin	Coconut and Berry Smoothie Bowl
15	Protein-Packed Cottage Cheese Parfait	Lemon Pepper Baked Chicken Thighs	Lemon Pepper Baked Chicken Thighs	Roasted Red Pepper Hummus with Veggie Sticks
16	Mushroom and Spinach Breakfast Burrito	Pineapple Teriyaki Beef Skewers	Pineapple Teriyaki Beef Skewers	Walnut and Date Protein Bars
17	Cranberry Walnut Overnight Oats	Greek-Style Stuffed Bell Peppers with Ground Lamb	Greek-Style Stuffed Bell Peppers with Ground Lamb	Orange and Ginger Infused Watermelon Cubes
18	Tomato Basil Breakfast Sandwich	Honey Mustard Glazed Chicken Breasts	Honey Mustard Glazed Chicken Breasts	Greek Yogurt and Mixed Berry Popsicles
19	Greek Yogurt and Berry Pancake Stack	Spiced Orange Glazed Pork Loin	Spiced Orange Glazed Pork Loin	Spiced Pumpkin Seed Clusters

Day	Breakfast	Lunch	Dinner	Snack/Dessert
20	Southwest Quinoa Breakfast Skillet	Slow-Cooked Pulled Pork Tacos	Slow-Cooked Pulled Pork Tacos	Dark Chocolate Avocado Truffles
21	Pear and Walnut Breakfast Salad	Moroccan Spiced Lamb Kabobs	Moroccan Spiced Lamb Kabobs	Berry Blast Yogurt Parfait
22	Chickpea and Spinach Breakfast Hash	Tuscan Herb Roasted Chicken Thighs	Tuscan Herb Roasted Chicken Thighs	Cinnamon Apple Slices with Almond Butter
23	Orange and Pistachio Chia Pudding	Citrus Glazed Chicken Skewers	Citrus Glazed Chicken Skewers	Greek Yogurt and Honey Frozen Blueberry Bites
24	Turkey Sausage and Veggie Egg Cups	Cumin-Spiced Turkey Burgers with Avocado	Cumin-Spiced Turkey Burgers with Avocado	Avocado Chocolate Mousse
25	Banana Nut Overnight Oats	Basil Pesto Chicken with Roasted Vegetables	Basil Pesto Chicken with Roasted Vegetables	Roasted Chickpeas with Smoky Paprika
26	Pesto and Tomato Breakfast Wrap	Grilled Lemon Herb Chicken Breasts	Grilled Lemon Herb Chicken Breasts	Almond and Chia Seed Energy Bites

Day	Breakfast	Lunch	Dinner	Snack/Dessert
27	Cacao and Almond Butter Smoothie	Rosemary Balsamic Roasted Turkey	Rosemary Balsamic Roasted Turkey	Baked Sweet Potato Chips with Rosemary
28	Veggie-Packed Breakfast Burrito Bowl	Cranberry-Orange Glazed Veal	Cranberry-Orange Glazed Veal	Mango Salsa with Whole Grain Pita Chips
29	Coconut Chia Seed Pudding Parfait	Lamb Patties with Cilantro and Spices	Lamb Patties with Cilantro and Spices	Vanilla Chia Pudding with Fresh Berries
30	Apple Cinnamon Walnut Breakfast Bowl	Citrus Glazed Chicken Skewers	Teriyaki Glazed Pineapple Salmon	Dark Chocolate Avocado Truffles

This is a general layout; you can customize it further based on individual preferences, dietary needs, and calorie requirements. Always consult with a healthcare professional or a nutritionist before entering into this diet.

CONCLUSION

Congratulations on starting this journey toward a healthier lifestyle with the DASH Diet! By choosing nutrient-rich foods, embracing a balance of flavors, and making conscious decisions about your dietary intake, you've taken a significant step toward supporting your overall well-being.

Remember, the DASH Diet isn't just a temporary fix; it's a sustainable approach to healthy eating. As you've explored the diverse range of recipes in this cookbook, you've witnessed the delicious possibilities that align with the principles of this heart-healthy diet.

Every meal is an opportunity to nourish your body and delight your taste buds. From vibrant breakfast bowls to savory dinners and delightful desserts, you've discovered how enjoyable and fulfilling wholesome eating can be.

We encourage you to continue experimenting with these recipes, adapting them to your taste preferences and lifestyle. The DASH Diet is not about restriction but about finding joy in making choices that benefit your health.

Your feedback is invaluable! We'd love to hear about your experiences with the recipes and how they've positively impacted your health journey. Share your thoughts, suggestions, and your favorite creations. Your feedback fuels our commitment to providing you with the best tools for a healthier, more vibrant life.

Thank you for choosing the DASH Diet. Here's to your health, happiness, and the many more delicious and heart-healthy meals that await you!

Sincerely,

Emma Willson

P.S. If you have a moment, please leave us a review. Your insights help us continually improve and inspire others to embrace a healthier lifestyle. Scan the QR code in the listing using your smartphone's camera or QR code scanner app.

Thank you!

21-Day Blood Pressure Monitoring Card

Day	Morning BP (mmHg)	Evening (mmHg)	Notes
Day 1			
Day 2			
Day 3			
Day 4			
Day 5			
Day 6			
Day 7			
Day 8			
Day 9			
Day 10			
Day 11			
Day 12			
Day 13			
Day 14			
Day 15			
Day 16			
Day 17			
Day 18			
Day 19			
Day 20			
Day 21			

Instruction

- Measure your blood pressure twice a day, in the morning and evening.
- Record the values in the corresponding columns.
- Note any relevant details or activities that might impact your blood pressure.
- Consult with your healthcare professional if you notice consistent high or low readings.

BONUS2

Welcome to the bonus chapter of our DASH Diet cookbook, dedicated to incorporating physical activities into your daily routine. Staying active is a crucial aspect of maintaining a healthy lifestyle, and these chair exercises are designed to make fitness accessible to everyone, regardless of fitness level or mobility. Remember to consult with your healthcare provider before starting any new exercise routine.

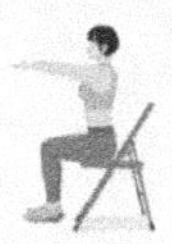 Sit on a chair with your feet firmly planted on the floor at a 90-degree angle. Extend your arms forward and perform circular motions with your wrists in both directions. Next, open your arms in different directions, ensuring that your palms face down.

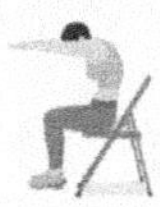 Transition to step 2 by maintaining the position from step 1 but rounding your back. Make rotational movememt with your arms as if you were swimming.

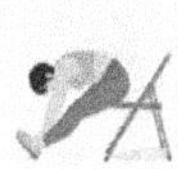 Move to step 3 by leaning your body forward, extending your toes, and holding for a few seconds. Ensure you maintain a neutral head position without lowering it down.

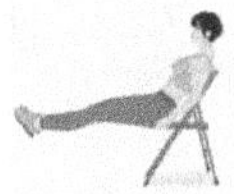 For step 4, sit on the edge of the chair, lean your body backward, and extend your legs forward. Hold this position briefly. If challenging, perform the exercise alternately on each leg.

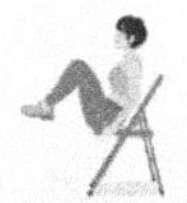 In step 5, sit up straight, lift your legs towards your chest, and lower them without touching the floor. Optionally, alternate between legs.

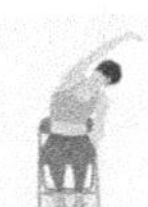 Maintain an upright position for step 6, tilting your torso gently to the left and right while keeping your back fixed. Perform controlled bends to stretch your muscles.

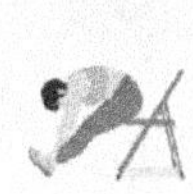 Finally, for step 7, relax by leaning your body forward, rounding your back, and ensuring your head remains unflexed.

Conclusion:
Incorporating these chair exercises into your routine can improve flexibility, strength, and overall well-being. Remember to listen to your body, modify the exercises as needed, and enjoy the benefits of staying active. As always, consult with your healthcare provider before starting a new exercise program, especially if you have any existing health concerns. We hope you find these exercises both enjoyable and beneficial!